TABLE OF CONTENTS

What is a Yoga Wall?

The yoga rope wall is a series of ropes, and sometimes slings, attached to a wall in different ways and used as a yoga prop. This protocol was originally used by Yoga teacher BKS Iyengar to assist students in finding better alignment and improving their yoga practice, as well as daily life. The wall has evolved in many ways over the years, and alternate variations exist in the fitness community in the form of suspension training and even, to some degree, Barre classes.

Traditional models utilized ropes and handles attached to the wall at varying heights. Ropes were tied into loops with handles and utilized to hold as students moved into a posture, hanging or pulling on the rope to assist in further development of the pose. Today's yoga wall often consists of the same equipment, but sometimes other attachments, such as pelvic inversion slings and elastic bands, are used for different purposes and comfort.

The practice, sometimes referred to as Yoga Karunta, can be a wonderful place for beginners and those with disabilities to experience depth in a more supported way, and can also be used by advanced practitioners to create more opening and understanding in progressions. It can be used to deepen stretches, but it can also be used to help strengthen the core and other parts of the body.

While there are some formal Yoga Wall building companies out there, one can use simple solutions that drape over a door or attach to a chin up bar in many circumstances. This book will demonstrate inexpensive ways to create one for yourself. It is recommended that you contact a contractor to install one in your home, and a structural engineer if you plan to put one in your studio. If you plan to put several people on your yoga wall at once, you must make certain that your wall can support the weight and dynamics of the exercises.

Who can benefit from use of a yoga wall?

Anyone!

The yoga wall assists people in poses – even in chairs! It helps to enhance stretches, understand alignment, develop strength, and promote body awareness. There really are no limits to what you can do with it, and this book hopes to offer just an introduction. Exploring on your own will help you to develop your practice in Yoga Karunta.

I have used the yoga wall to help students with multiple sclerosis to find more awareness in balance in a safe, supported way. Many people with back pain (please make certain they do not have any contraindications to a regular yoga practice before utilizing this modality with them) have found relief with some of the exercises outlined in the next chapters. Students have found strength in their legs, core and upper body. Used wisely, some people can perform stretches that are difficult to attain on the floor due to knee or hip issues.

Those in athletic condition can benefit from the deeper stretches and understanding of their bodies, as well as fun core exercises that will certainly challenge even the most agile among us.

Because it is a wall, it is not difficult to design stretching exercises that might benefit those who are wheelchair bound.

Kids LOVE the yoga wall. Hanging upside-down can be a fantastic way to calm them as well as help them build self-confidence.

Many of the poses can be useful for prenatal clients, allowing them gentle relief from back pain and sciatica.

Even older students can keep themselves limber and find better balance with some of the exercises.

Safety

While all the general rules of yoga and fitness will apply – such as being aware of one's limits and abilities, there are one or two other concerns when using the rope wall.

Always check your ropes and slings to make sure they are attached well and there are no parts of concern in installation. It is a good idea to get into the habit of checking them before each use. Check the ropes for fray or loose knots. Check the attachments to the wall itself to make certain there is no movement. If you are using carabiners, check to make sure they are properly closed (and of strong weight). Common sense precautions will prevent catastrophe.

Always keep tension on the ropes or slings. When getting in and out of any position, never allow slack onto the rope. You have to learn to trust the wall and that it will hold you. If you don't, this is a pointless series of exercises. The main reason to use the wall is to allow it to support you to fall deeper into the pose.

As a general rule of thumb, make sure participants are grounded at the wall. Many people will try to work the poses with their feet away from the wall. They are far more effective, not to mention safer, if they ground their foot or feet into the wall for security. This way they won't be pulled back by the ropes and swing into the wall. Some poses may involve walking the feet up the wall. Please avoid this except where absolutely necessary. While it can be fun to do, many newer practitioners will slip and cause possible injury to themselves or others. Most poses (baring one or two) can be done with the feet against the wall and the floor. This is optimal as they are supported on more than one level and there is no chance of slipping. Again, there are one or two poses where it will be necessary, however if there is another option, always use it.

Body mechanics are very important in this practice, so never allow a student or yourself to put too much stress on the joints. It is easy to allow the weight to go into a shoulder that is just a little too open and exposed or a hip to go farther than it should because of the ropes. Always be aware of your limitations and remind students not to go past theirs. As with all yoga, a little discomfort can be good but pain is always bad.

Building Your Wall

There are many options you can utilize to build your yoga wall. As I advised before, it would be best to have a contractor help you install any variation, except the door option. Many ideas can be found on the internet with pictures and even diagrams.

In general, but not exclusively, the ropes are hung at 82", 40", and 18" from the floor. They are set at a standard 25" apart (the exact distance of the studs in the wall it is hanging on). There are many, many diagrams available online and for purchase if you plan to build your own, or have one built.

There are also companies that make pre-fabricated yoga walls such as The Great Yoga Wall. They still need to be installed, however they offer a template for installation that most carpenters can follow. The benefit of this type wall is they have pre-fabricated attachments that allow for easy changing of ropes, handles, slings, Pilates foot apparatus and springs, barres, and probably many other attachments I don't know about. It's a more expensive option, but they do make a beautiful product offer easier transition between different types of exercises.

The wall I have that is pictured in this book was made by a carpenter who followed the specifications on the website www.sandieyga.com/resources/ropewall . The carpenter made the handle holes round and put rope lighting behind the platform wall so it looks extra beautiful and is a real point of interest in our space. There are no absolute rules, however the general specifications are there for a reason.

The rope length for the ropes can vary to some degree, but in general the high ropes will land somewhere near the lower handle attachments. This can vary according to height of the practitioner. It's not necessarily exact, however the length you use should match for the set. If they are slightly off, you can remedy that by giving the longer rope a couple of twists. The lower ropes are generally shorter, often called short ropes. Consequently, it may sometimes be useful to put long ropes on the low handles and short ropes on the high handles for various reasons. It may also be useful to tie a yoga strap on any of the ropes to make it longer, as for use in a chair.

The ropes are generally climbing grade ropes. These can be bought online or at a sporting goods store. We use a lot of climbing gear on the yoga wall.

There are many directions on YouTube on how to tie the ropes, however it is generally a fisherman's knot. You can buy pre-made ropes at ToolsForYoga.com or YogaProps.com. I use yoga straps for my low ropes, mainly because I had them available and did not like the way the ropes felt in the poses.

The high ropes can be pulled together to make a sling; however, most people find that uncomfortable. I prefer to have a pelvic inversion sling for this purpose. They can be purchased online at several shops, however shop around to make sure you get one that is affordable as well as easy to change the height of. There are several exercises utilizing the inversion sling at different heights in this book – and they are all fan favorites. Consequently, I have recently seen people using aerial hammocks on the wall as an inversion sling. This option is great, however may be difficult to adjust.

The slings I have are attached to the handles with carabiners. The carabiners move, so just be aware of that. Always make sure they are secure and locked. This is only the way I have installed them. If you have another way that works better for you, use it. Just remember, the sling should be adjustable in order to perform the different exercises outlined in this book.

Here is a photo of a homemade version at a friend's house. She used Sturdy handles mounted into the studs.

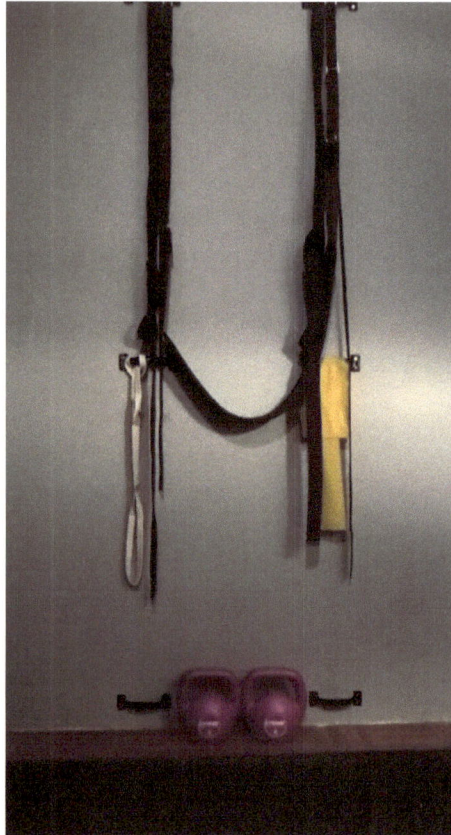

If you want to start inexpensively and not mount anything into the wall, using the door is a great way to go. The inversion sling I have, a Mysore Yoga Strap, can be mounted on the top of a closed door, similar to the below pictures of the rest of the equipment. All you need is a closed door and a little room!

For the High ropes, I found this suspension training kit at WalMart for less than $20.

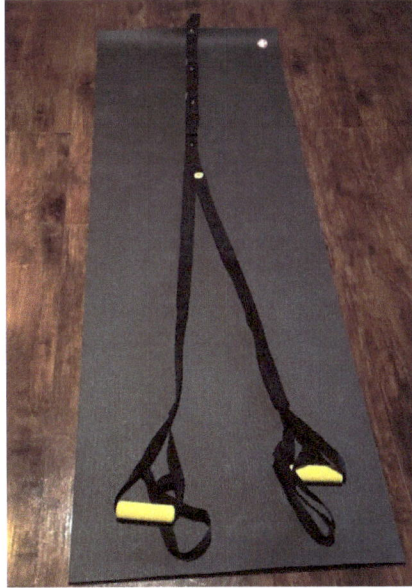

It goes over the door like this.

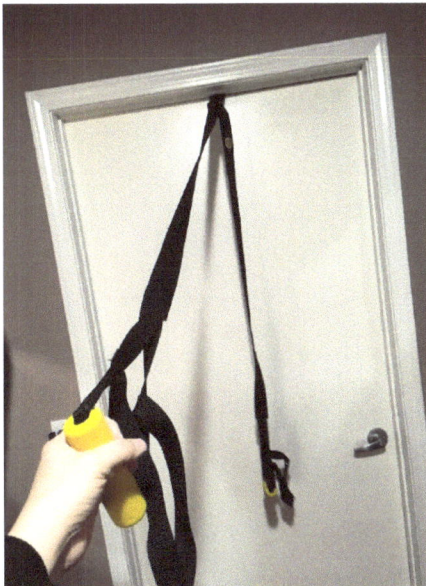
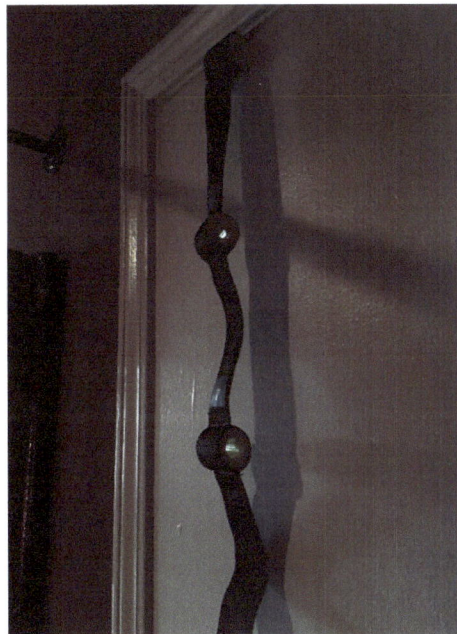

The low ropes can be easily made from two yoga straps, which can be bought at WalMart or online for less than $10. I recommend the smaller ones and the ones with buckles, not D rings as they will stay put for this better. They install like this:

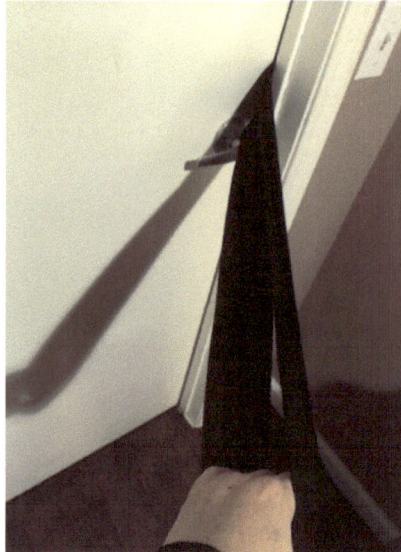

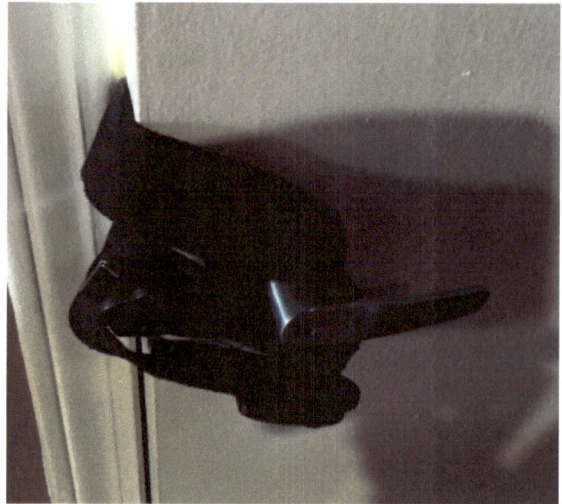

And for the low low ropes, just install them like this.

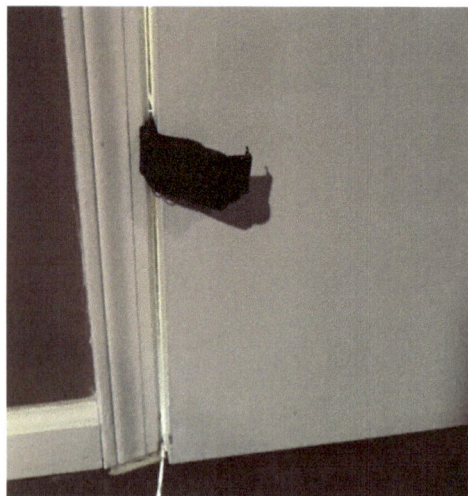

THE EXERCISES

Here I will outline several exercises, along with photos. I have separated them into categories, however they do not all fit perfectly into these categories Some may be in more than one place as it may fit into more than one category.

It is helpful to think through your session and try to group certain similar exercises together to help with flow. This is especially true if you are using the slings as they can be bothersome to adjust for different exercises. Keeping them at one height until it's time to move on will make life a little easier, in the long run.

When devising a protocol for a class or session, I will think of one or two areas I want to focus on – hip openers or backbends, say. I will think through what exercises will best accomplish this and set out to find a logical sequence for those goals.

It is helpful to know that sessions do not have to be exclusive to the wall. I will often teach a regular class and then bring them to the wall for some workshop style poses. I also sometimes offer a "Walls and Wheels" class that uses the yoga wheel for part of the class and the wall for another part. It's all up to you to decide how to use it.

High Ropes

Warm ups

These warm ups are combinations of some of the exercises you may find further in this book. They are mainly to be used for a sole wall workout, or if you are using the wall first. They are to be done with the breath, not holding anything for too long and allowing for the body to build some heat.

Squats

Take hold of the high ropes. Make sure they are even. Walk back until there is tension in the ropes.

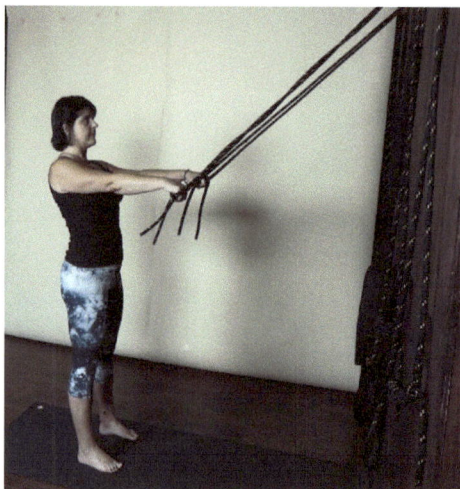

Put your weight back into your heels and sit back into a squat.

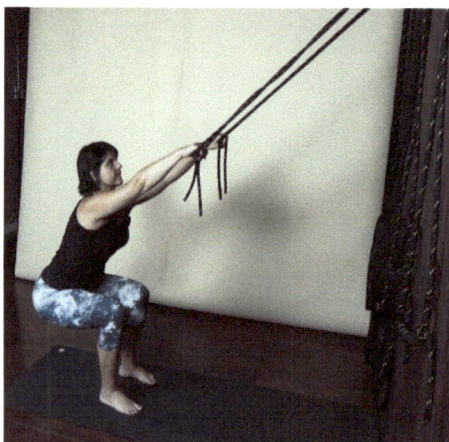

Make sure you are sitting back and not leaning into your toes. The ropes help with this if you make sure you are pulling back with your arms long. It may be helpful for newer students or those with any disabiity to have a chair or stool behind them to sit back to. This will help them to establish their awarness in the pose and be less fearful of sitting back.

Stand back up using all four corners of the feet to press and lift.

Repeat 8-10 times.

Repeat the sequence with feet apart and turned out as well as crossing one foot over knee (or lifting it forward), or even eagle wrapping the leg. Choose at least three variations and do 8-10.

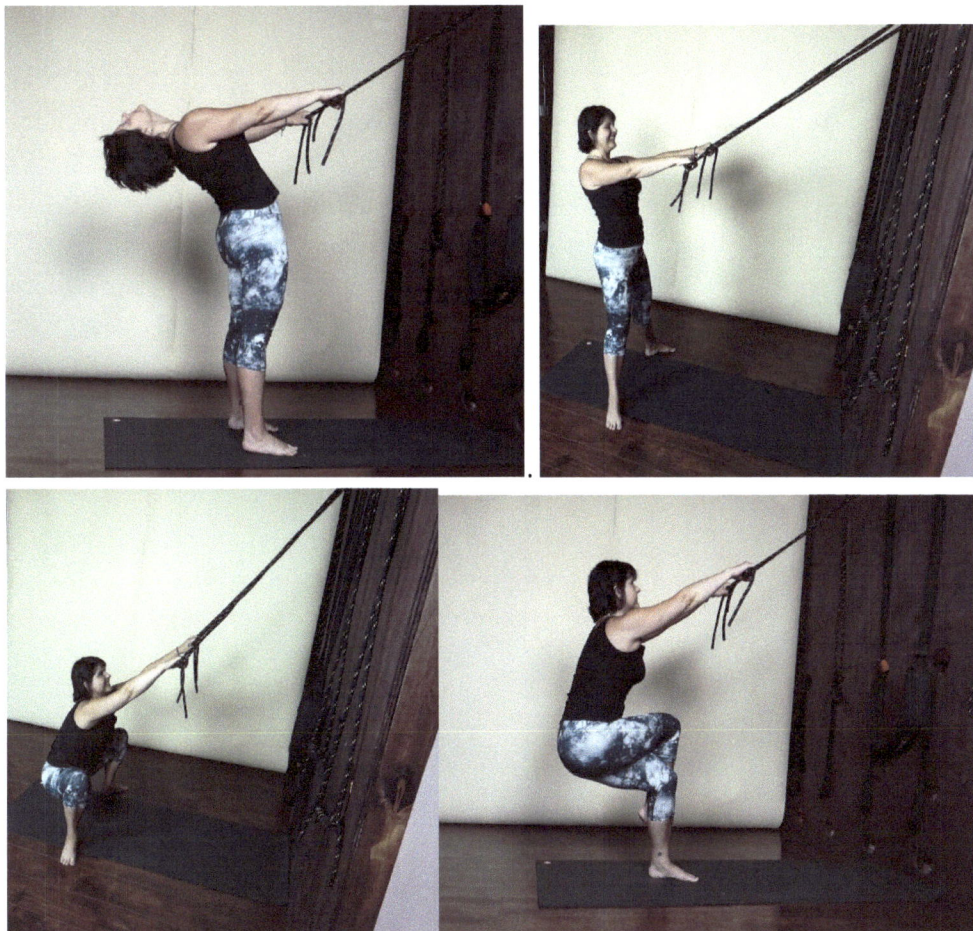

In between sets or even in between squats one can take a backbend by standing up and falling back, lifting the chest and pushing the hips forward. Remember to draw the shoulders down and slightly rotate them open for the best effect.

Arm Openers

Using the High ropes, take hold and walk away from the wall facing away. Open the arms into a cross. Don't let the arms be pulled back enough to put stress on the shoulders. Keep the chest and core engaged and don't allow the back to arch forward. Keep the chest lifted.

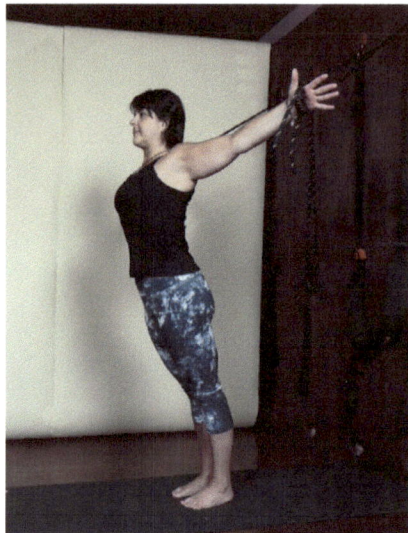

Next, allow the body to reach from side to side, keeping both hips fixed forward and allowing the lowering arm to reach back. Keep the chest engaged and the core strong. Don't allow the arms to move separately from the body. The entire upper body moves as one unit.

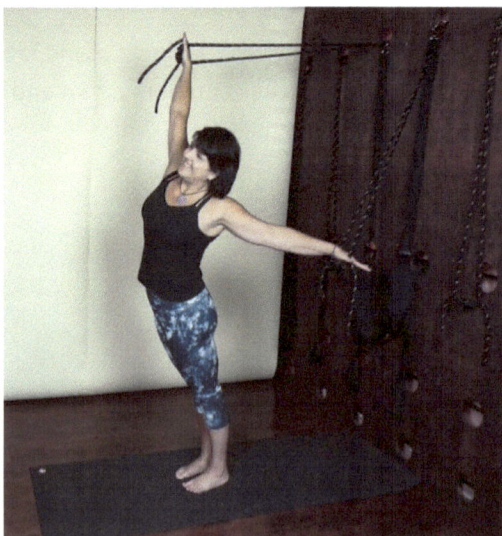

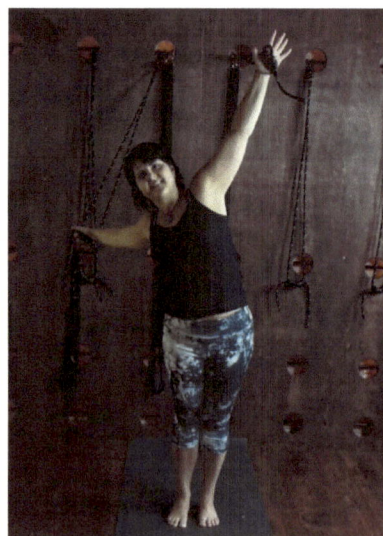

A Tricep stretch can be nice here. Hold both ropes in both hands and draw the elbows up above your head. Let the hands slightly bend back.

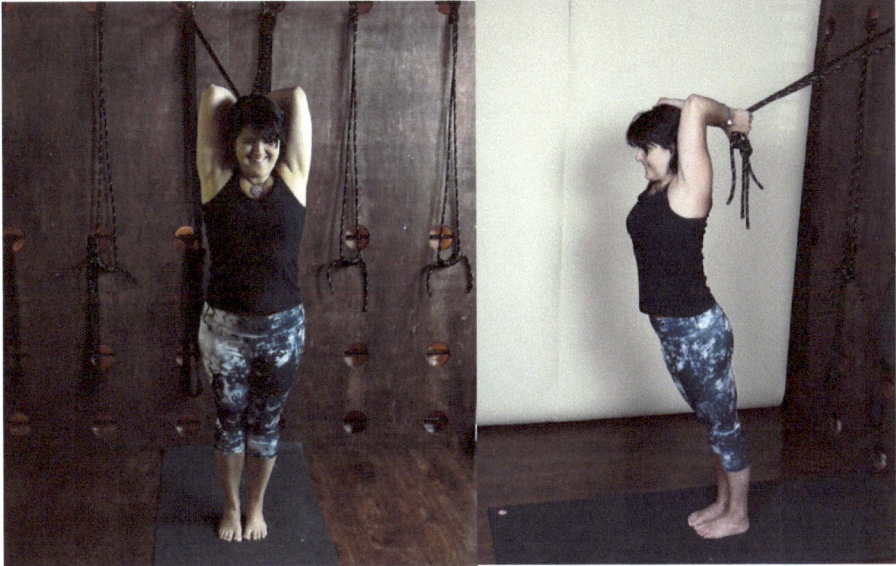

Sun Salutations

**The following exercises are not advisable for those with shoulder injuries.*

Walk away from the wall with your hands holding the high ropes. Draw your arms back, with hands rotating inward. Put some weight into the hands, leaning forward. Keep weight in the ropes as you walk back to the wall with feet on the wall into a forward fold. Note that the bottom is away from the wall and the body weight is in the ropes.

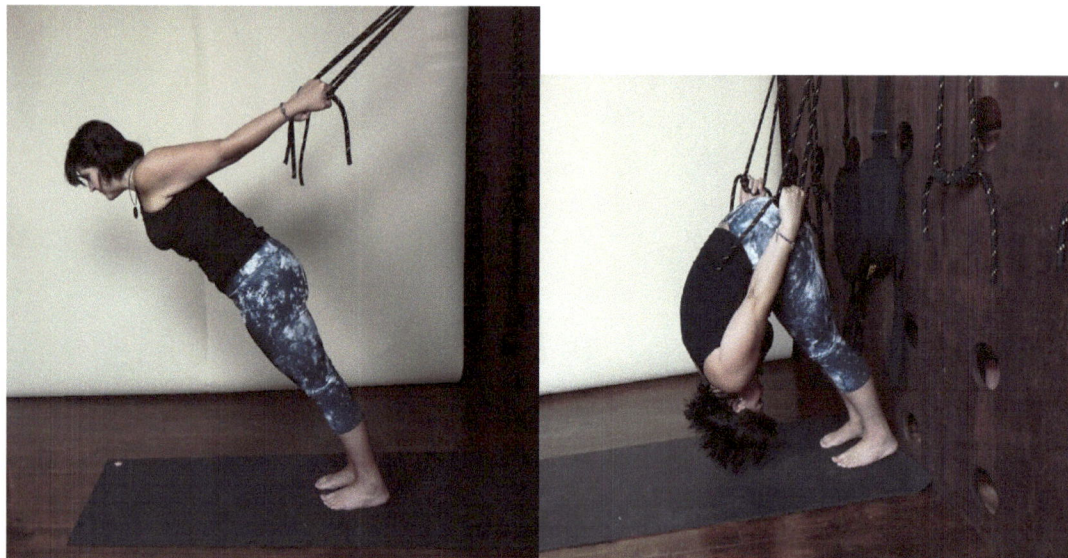

Slowly press out away from the wall to lengthen the torso out into an upward dog variation. PLEASE NOTE: you will need to turn the hands open as you move forward. You will not go into a deep backbend in this variation.

Pull back to forward fold then back out. Use the breath, inhale as you lengthen, exhale as you contract.

Remember to rotate the shoulders as you move so as not to put more stress on them.

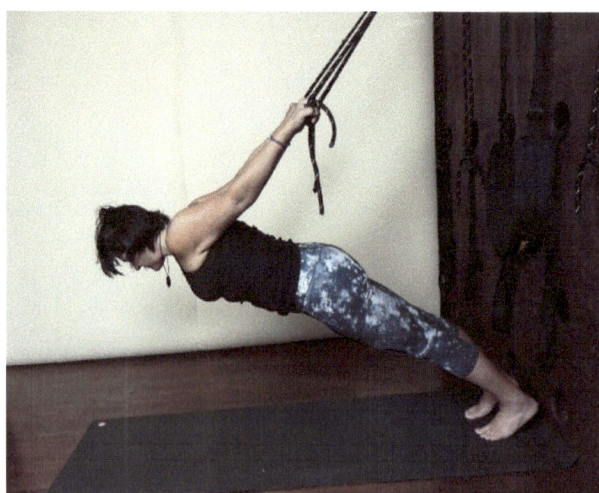

Keep weight in hands to walk forward and release.

Shoulder Stretch

***As in the previous exercise, this stretch is not advisable for shoulder injuries.

Face the wall and hold the high ropes. Swim your arms open as you come to a forward bend, lifting the arms behind you. For a deeper stretch, walk back a little or lean into your heels/hips.

Make certain that you are steady as the pull on your arms could topple you forward if you don't sit back.

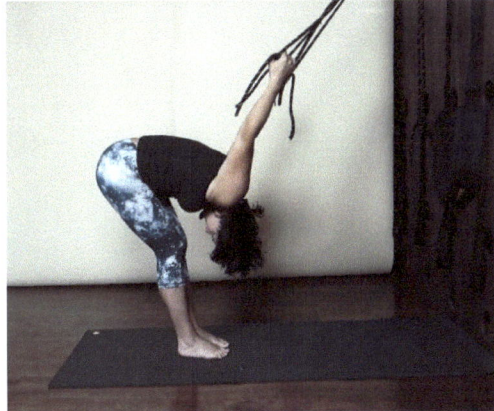

To make this deeper, start on your knees. Lean back for more intensity, forward for less.

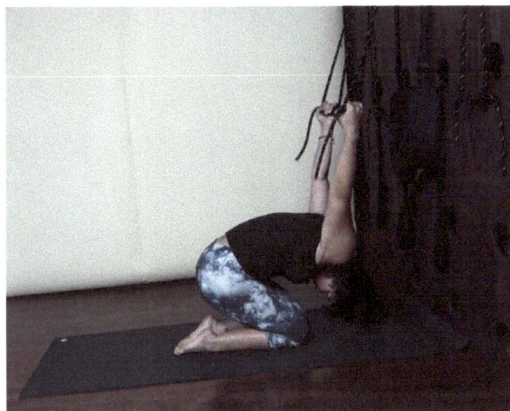

To come out, either let go or backwards swim your arms open and sit up.

Arm Exercises

Most of the arm exercises in this book are done using the high ropes. It's nice to use these combined with the arm and shoulder stretches, although holding onto the ropes can leave your hands tired and sore. It may be helpful to do these exercises, then switch to slings for a while then come back to do the stretches, or some variation.

A note about the angle of your body in these next few exercises: The closer you are to standing, the easier this is. If you lean back and put your feet closer to the wall, you have to work harder against gravity. By keeping your body as straight as possible, you will not only stabilize your core, but use your arms much more to do the work. Do each exercise 8-12 times.

High Rows

Stand facing the wall and grab the high ropes. Find tension in the ropes and lean back into them with long arms. Walk your feet towards the wall to the desired angle (closer to the wall is harder). Keeping your elbows high, pull back into them, squeezing your shoulders back. Slowly release. Repeat.

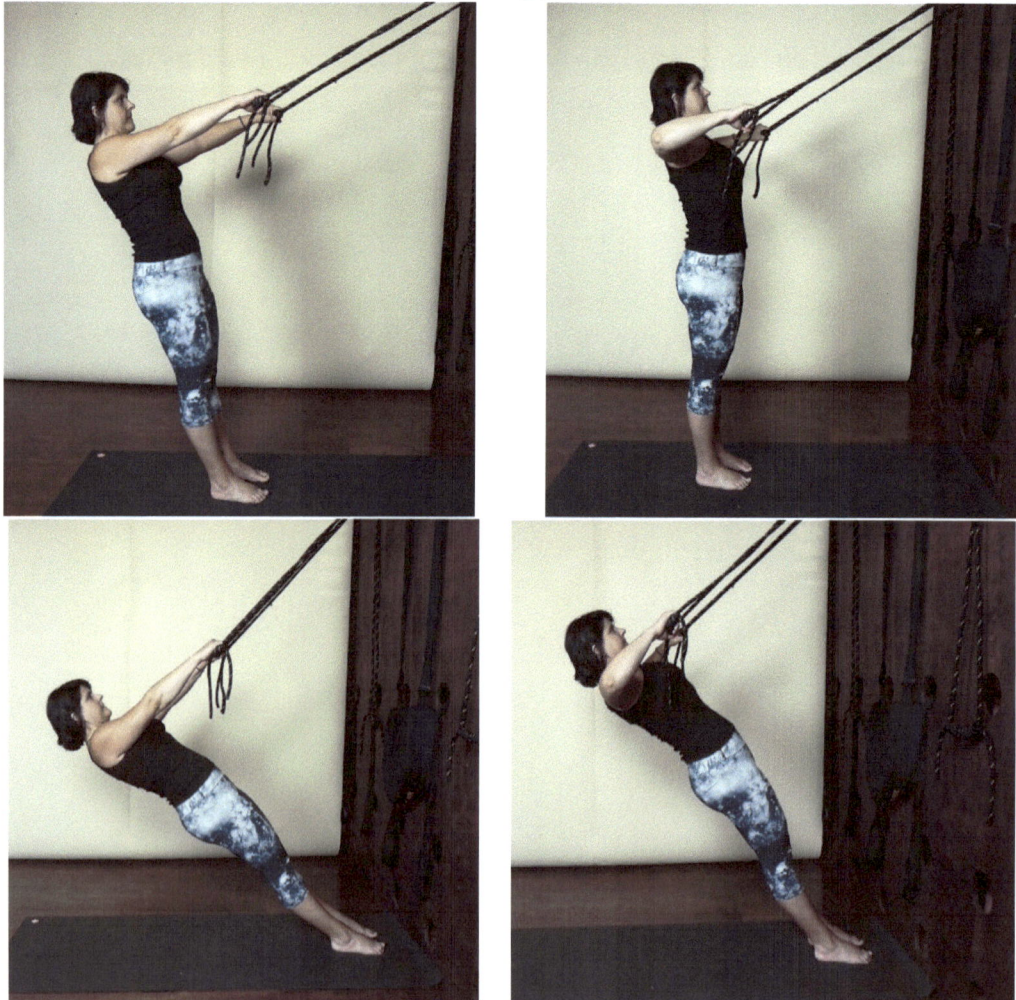

Low rows are the same, only keep he elbows down by your sides and pull to your low ribs.

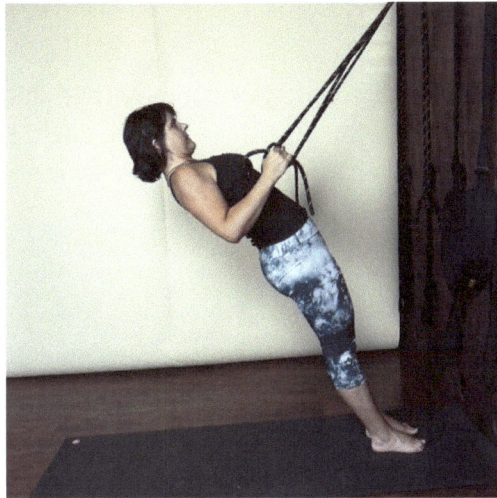

Bicep Curls

Extend the arms in front of you, palms facing up. Keep the elbows high (shoulder height) as you pull your hands towards your face. Slowly release and repeat. Keep the core solid, throughout.

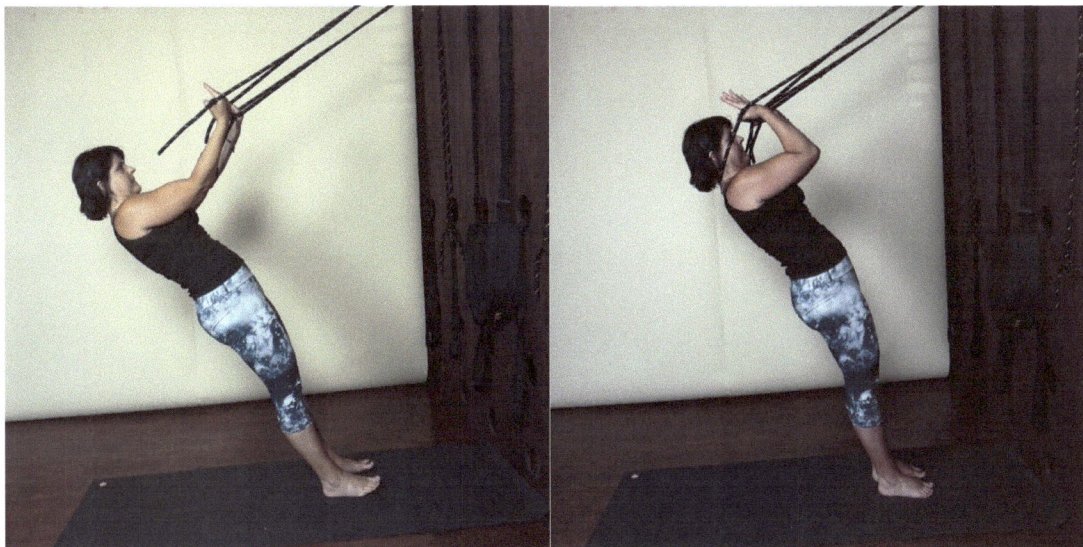

Bicep Pull-Up

Another great bicep exercise. Holding high ropes, walk o the wall and squat all the way down. Using the arms, pull yourself up as high as you can without pushing into the heels. Release down. Repeat. It may be helpful to put the knees into the wall for support. Try to use only the arm muscles if you can.

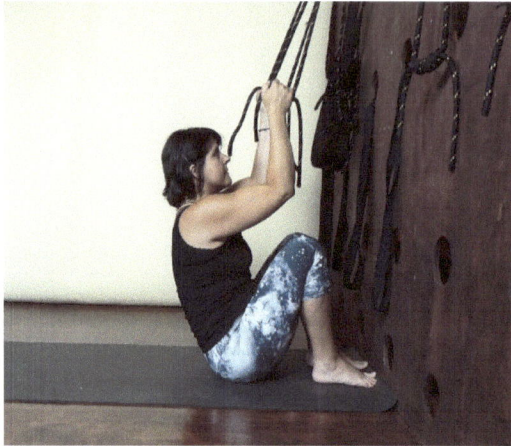

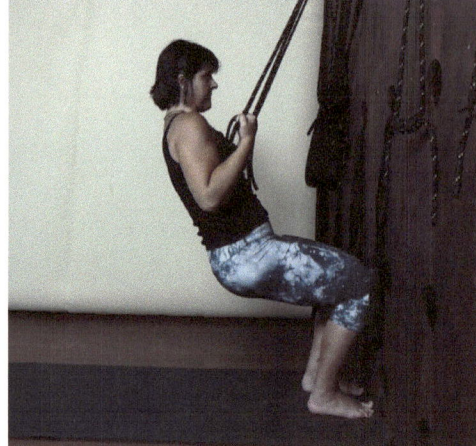

Tricep Press

We work the triceps a lot in yoga so I don't offer a lot here, however here is a nice tricep exercise.

Facing away from the wall, hold each high rope separately. Bring the arms overhead and walk out to get tension into the ropes. Walk your feet back towards the wall so that you are leaning into the ropes. Bend the elbows back, then puh into the hands, straighening them. Repeat. Keep the core strong and engaged.

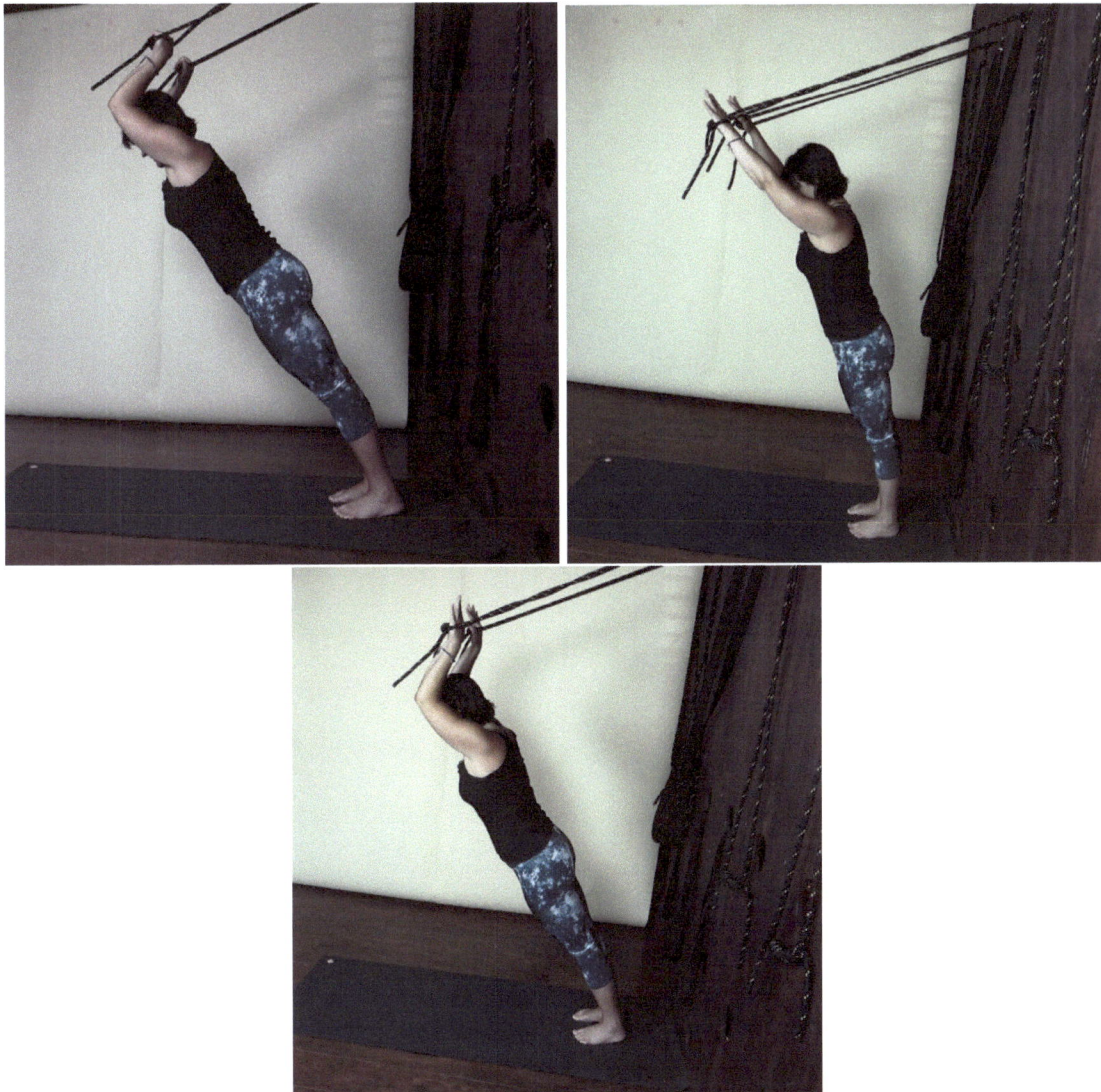

After all that arm work, this sure feels nice. Hold the handles, if you have them, and lean back, stretching the back out.

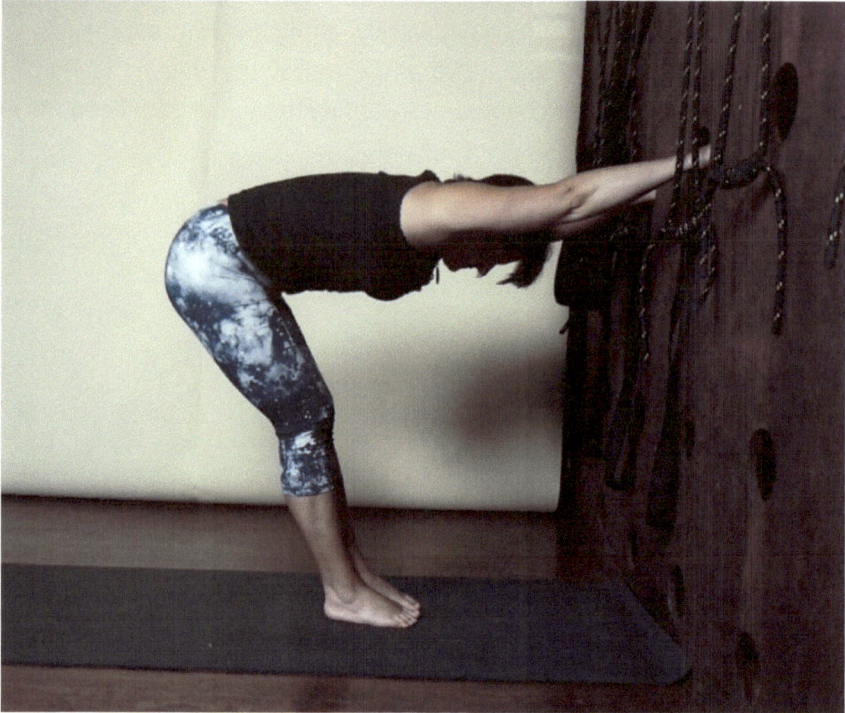

Traditional Standing Poses

I haven't included many of the traditional poses in this book, however there are variations of just about all of them. Here are a few with the high ropes.

These poses should be gotten into and worked in, breathing and experiencing the body, allowing it to open and feel the pose in a new way.

Warrior 1

Stand facing away from the wall. Place the back heel into the wall, turning the toes slightly forward. Hold the high ropes, not the handles, but high up. Step the front foot forward and come into your lunge, sliding down the ropes, keeping the arms long. Allow the upper body to be pulled into a slight backbend. Use the ropes to help work the upper body to face forward.

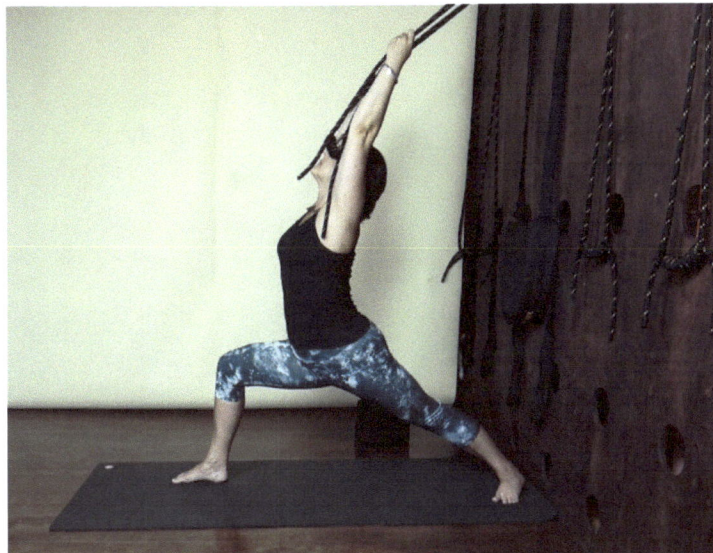

From Warrior 1, you can drop down to the back knee and work into a crescent. Holding the ropes allows for a deeper lunge and upper backbend. Pushing the back toes into the wall also helps!

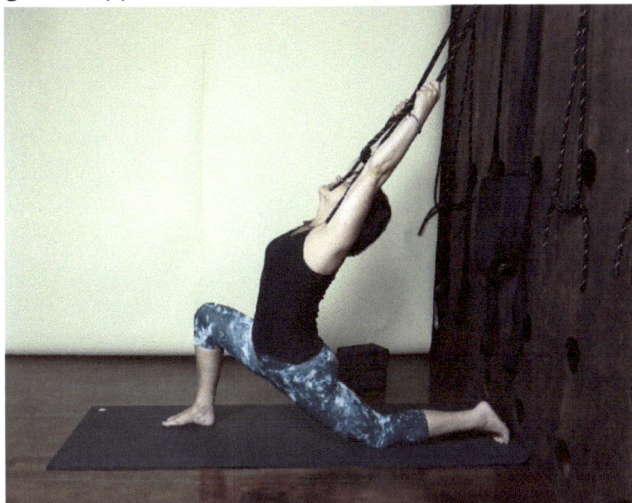

Warrior 2

Placing the back foot against the wall, side of the foot, grab hold of one or both high ropes. Hold them high up in the back hand – not at the handle. Walk the front foot out into poition, turning it away frm the wall. Come into your lunge, sliding the back hand down the rope with the arm long. Draw the front hand out. Notice how "hanging" on the rope allows you to deepen the lunge.

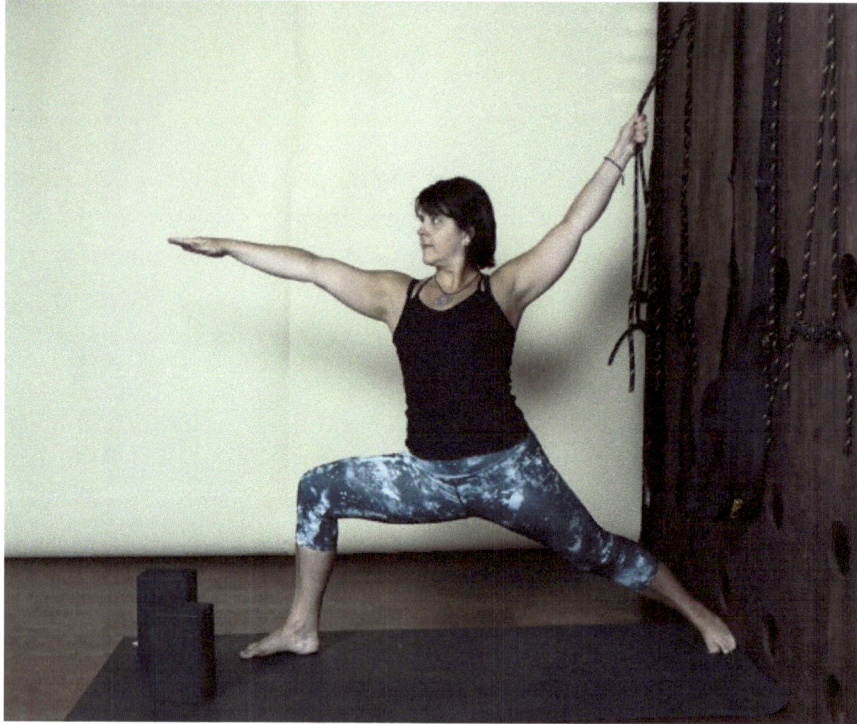

Reverse Warrior

From warrior 2, simply switch hands. It may be helpful to straighten the legs and reach high on the rope with the oposite hand, then slide back down into place.

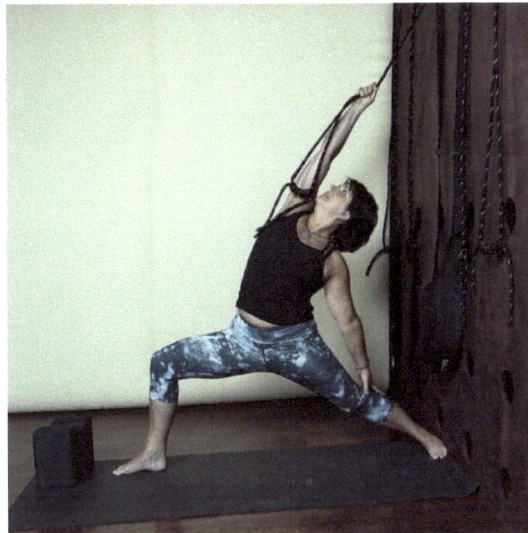

Extended Side Angle

Staying in Warrior 2 legs, holding the ropes with the wall hand, slide down to bring your opposite hand to the floor, block or elbow to knee. Notice how you can sink deeper into the lunge because you are not gripping in the hip to hold yourself. Reverse side angle is also a wonderful pose to try here. Come back up and twist to switch and hold the rope in the other hand. Bring the opposite hand down to the floor outside the knee/foot. This may challenge your balance a little bit and you may also have to lift into the toes of the back foot. To come out, simply let go.

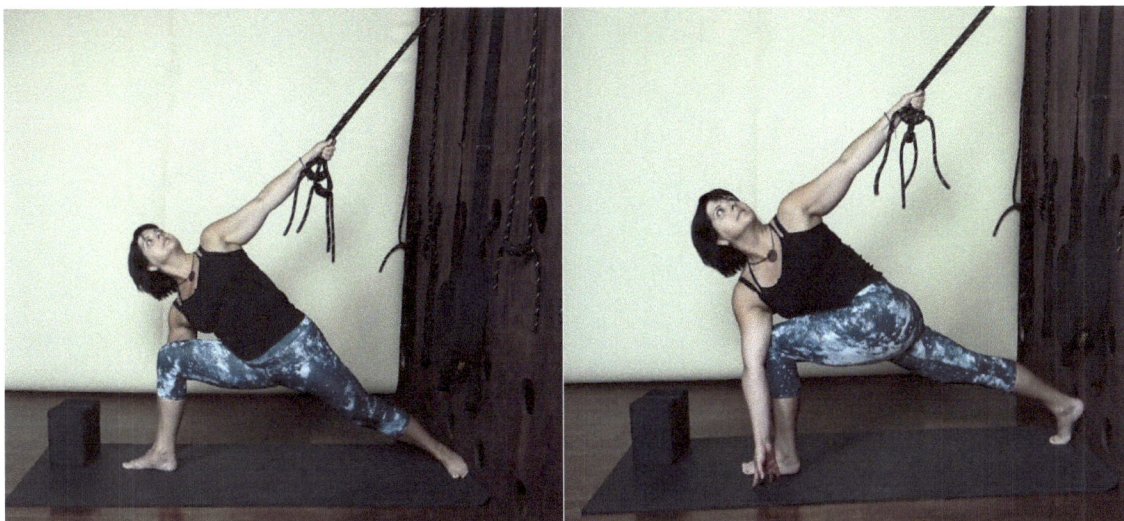

Triangle

Keeping the legs in the Warrior 2 stance, with back foot against the wall and the front foot out pointed away from it, Reach up and grab the ropes with the back hand. Working to keep the back hip and ribs (wall side) opening up, and keeping the torso very long, shift the hips slightly towards the wall as you reach forward with the arm and slide down the rope.

Keep both legs straight and draw the front leg back into the hip socket. Draw the front hand down. Using the ropes in this pose helps us to open up more. It may be helpful to reach for the ropes behind you, using your arm to pull you open more.

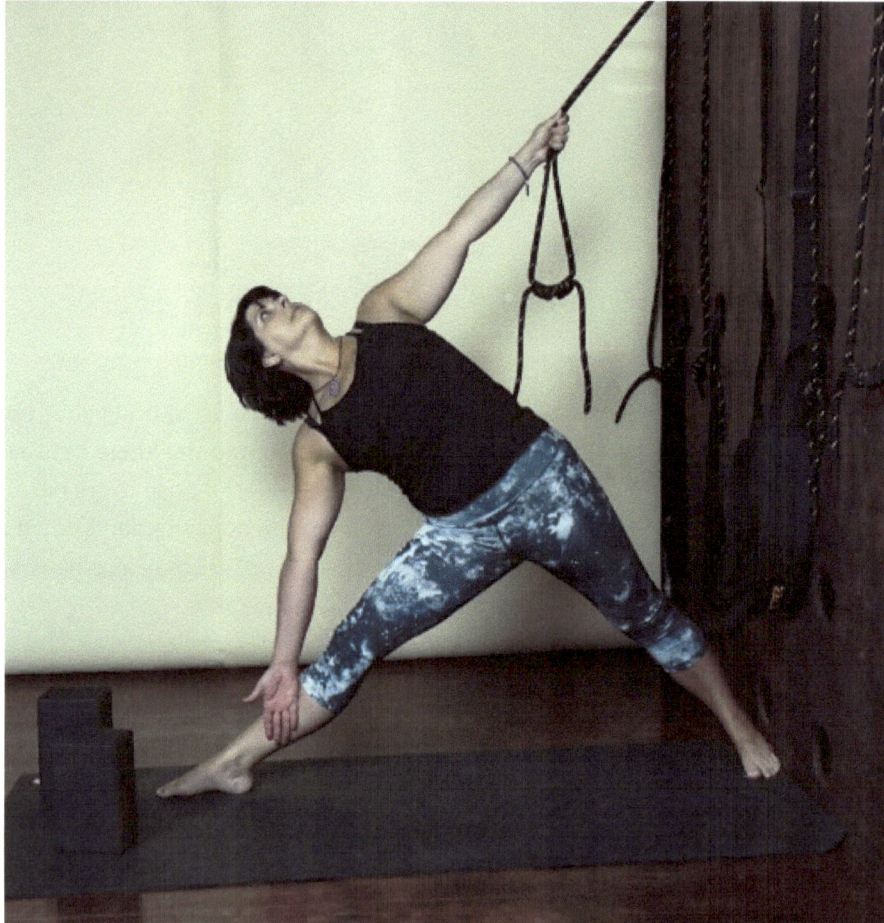

Standing Half Moon Pose

From Triangle pose, Standing Half Moon pose is just a matter of drawing your foot up to the wall, really. It may help to have a block the first time you try it so you have something to reach for, however you should be able to easily lift your hand off of it and play with other variations from there. When you are first trying this, make sure your back foot is really secure in the wall. After you feel steady and comfortable, maybe try to take the foot off and grab for it behind you.

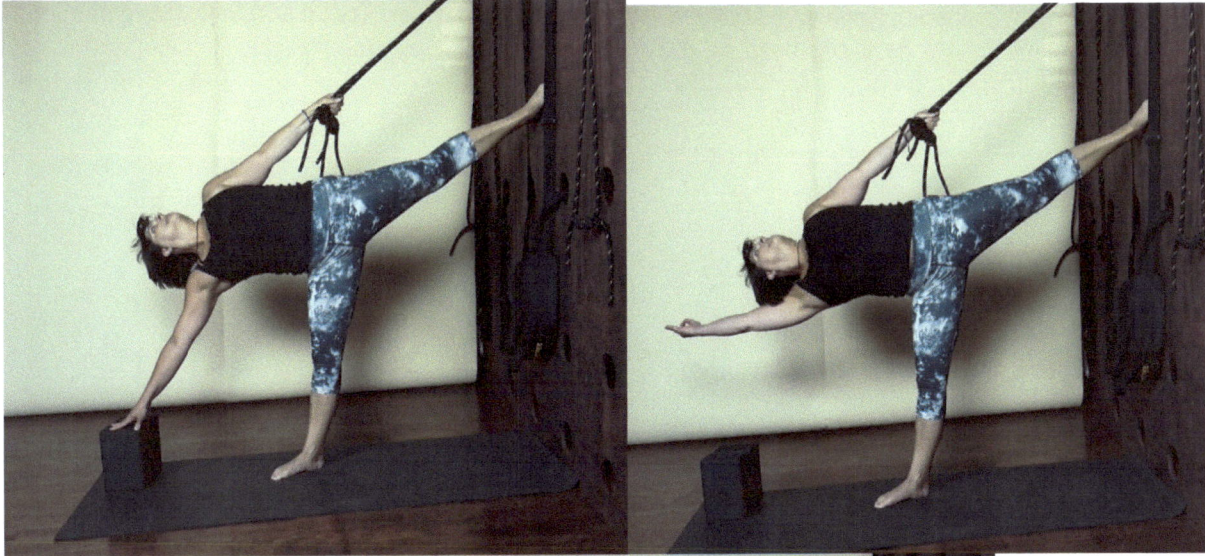

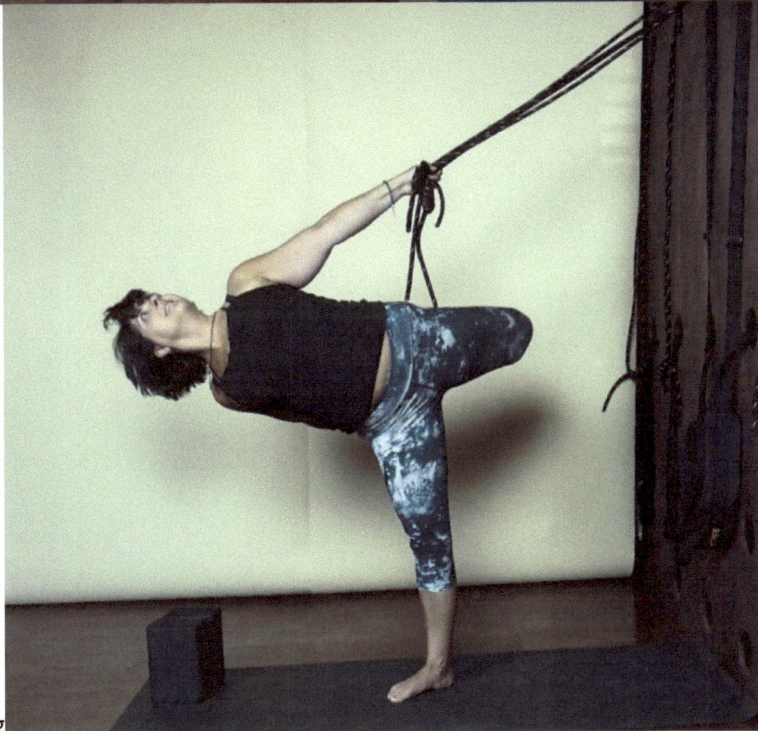

g

Side Plank Variation

Sit on your hip, both feet stacked, holding the handles of BOTH high ropes with the wall hand. Note: holding both ropes provides more stability.

Place the free hand on the floor. Press into your feet and the wall and lift the hips, hanging on the high ropes. If you cannot lift, try using a block under the low hand. Once you are up and feel strong enough, see if you can lift the low hand off the ground. You could also add some hip dips!

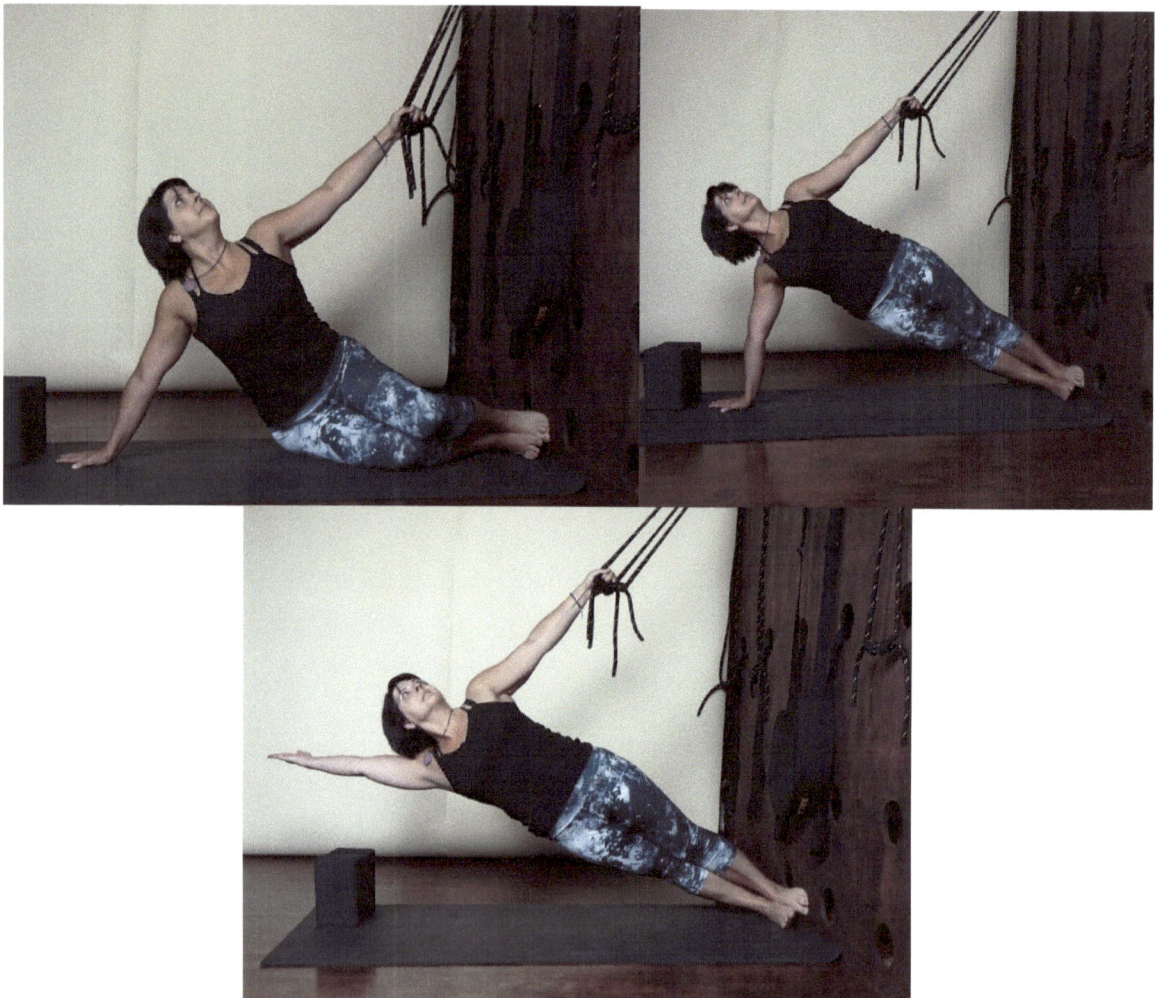

High ropes can also be used to aid with balance and backbends. Here are some balance variations to try that are great for those dealing with balance issues, aging populations and MS.

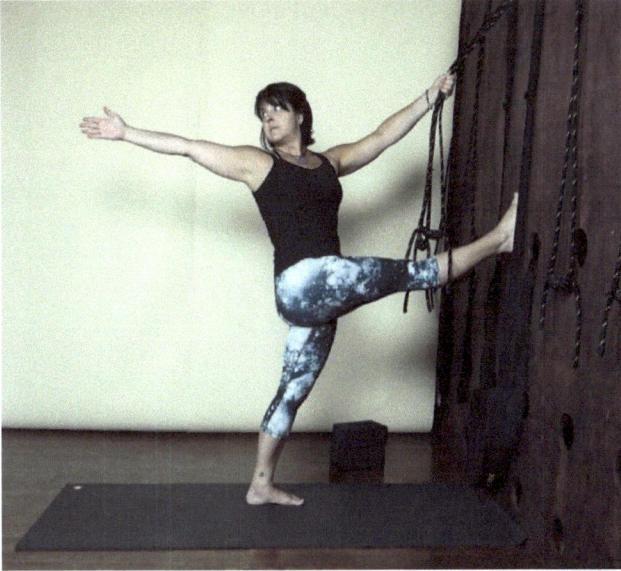

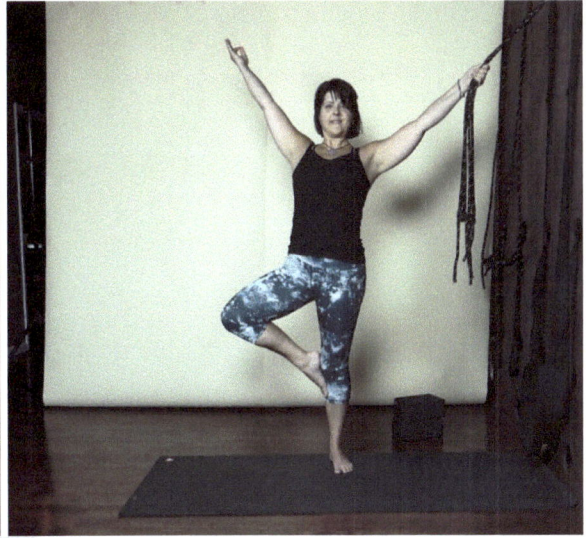

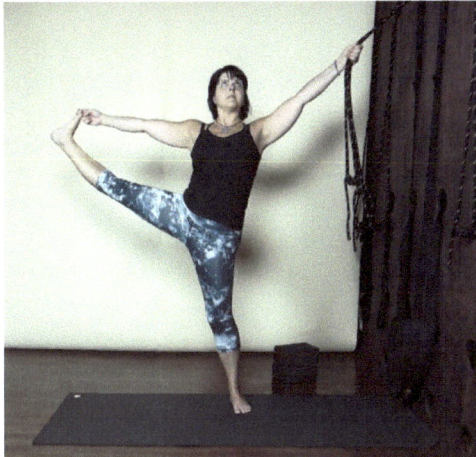

Deep Backbend

Start on the knees and slide forwards, dropping the hips as you move in. slide the hands down the ropes. It may be helpful to have a blanket under the knees.

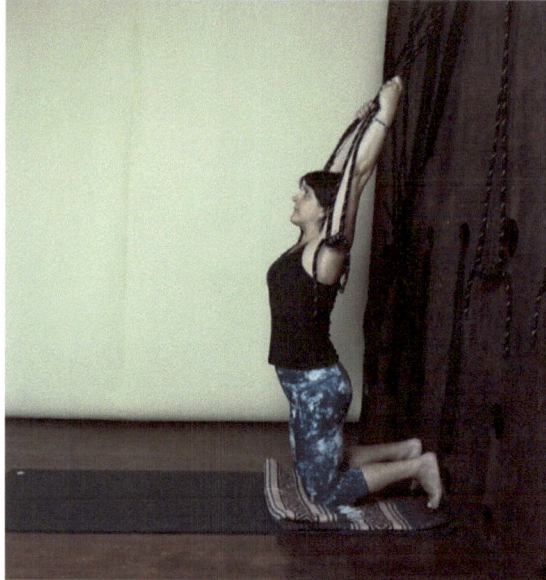

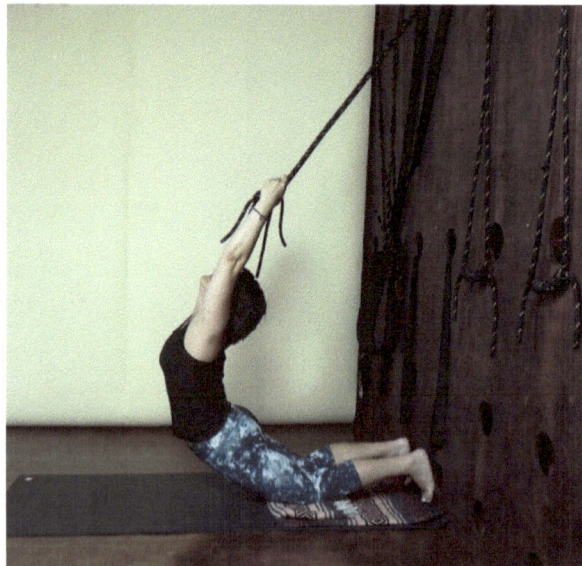

High Rope Core

High ropes can be used much like gymnastics rings in some respects. Here are a couple of exercises for the more acrobatic and daring.

Stand with your back against the wall. Hold the handles and press down. Lift your legs. Either lift and lower or hold.

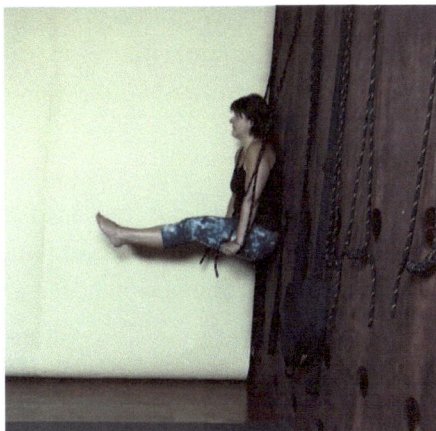

This one is fun, but challenging. Stand in frontof and facing the wall. Hold the low ropes as you walk forward, dropping into a forward fold (note this may be easier if you start on your knees). Lift the bottom up and lift one leg, then see if you can hang and hop the other leg up. I would make sure I was strong and up for the challenge. Also, you might want to test to make sure your head doesn't lay on the floor when you have your hands in the ropes – if you have longer arms this may not work unless you shorten the ropes.

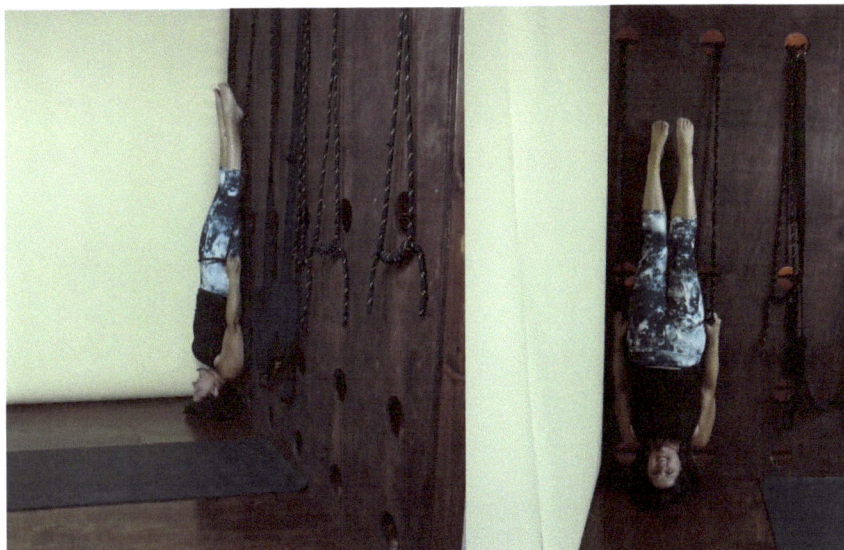

LOW ROPES

The low ropes offer several alignment- based exercises and will help most people better understand their hips. It will be helpful to have blocks, or even a chair for anyone who is particularly tight or dealing with an injury. The chair is not demonstrated in this book, however, you would generally place it in front of you instead of using blocks. You could then rest your elbows on it- or possibly the forehead, in some cases. Place the blocks or chair in front of you, within reach.

For the exercises in this series, we will put the ropes together to form a circle, then we will put ourselves into that circle. Place the ropes at your hip crease (when you draw your knee up off the ground the ropes sink into the fold). Walk your body weight out and lean into the tension.

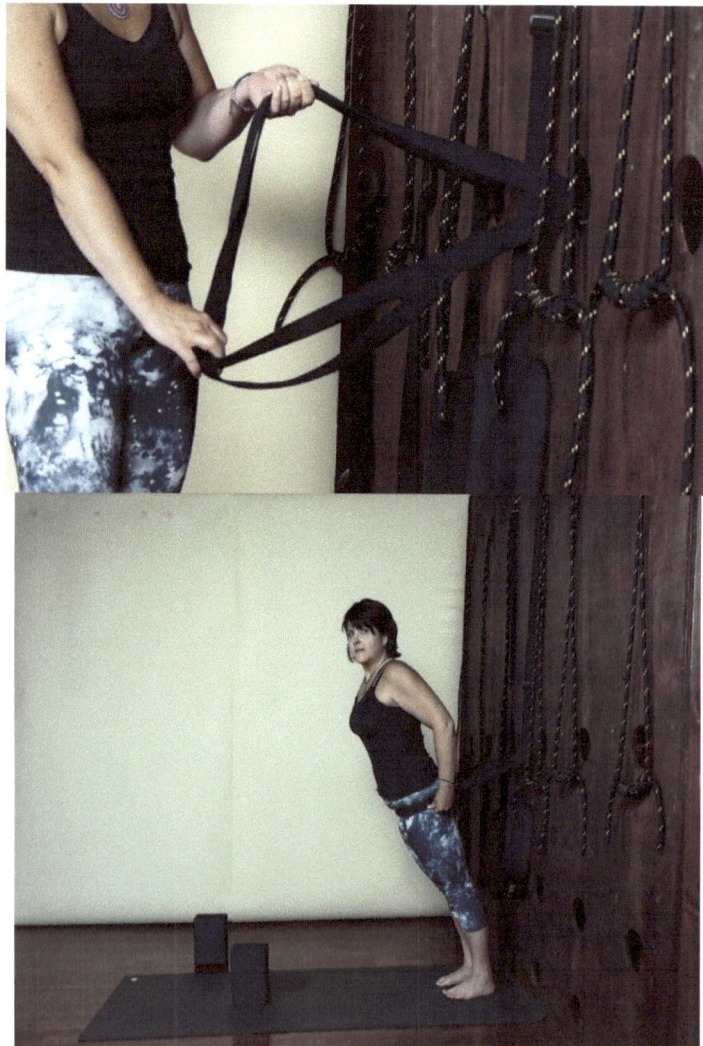

Reach forward and down. Place your hands on the blocks in the highest position. Walk your feet back to the wall.

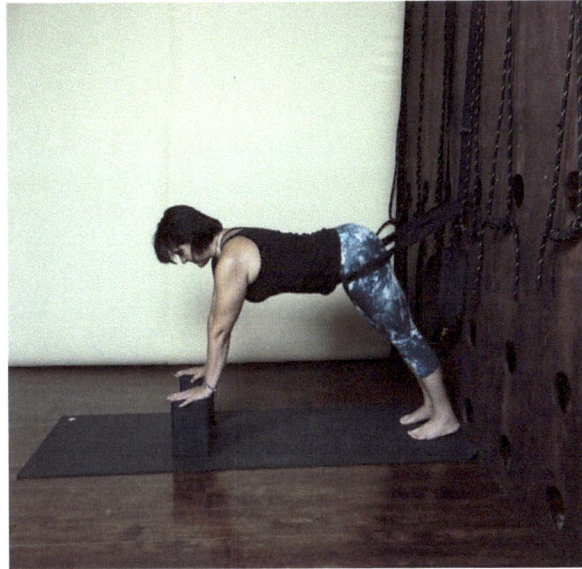

Downward Facing Dog

For most of us, we may want to keep the hands on the blocks until we are more open and we are nor rounding into the back in Downward Dog.

Keep the hands on the blocks in the high position, or work them down to the level that feels right and doesn't feel strain in the back. Draw the heels down and allow the head to hang.

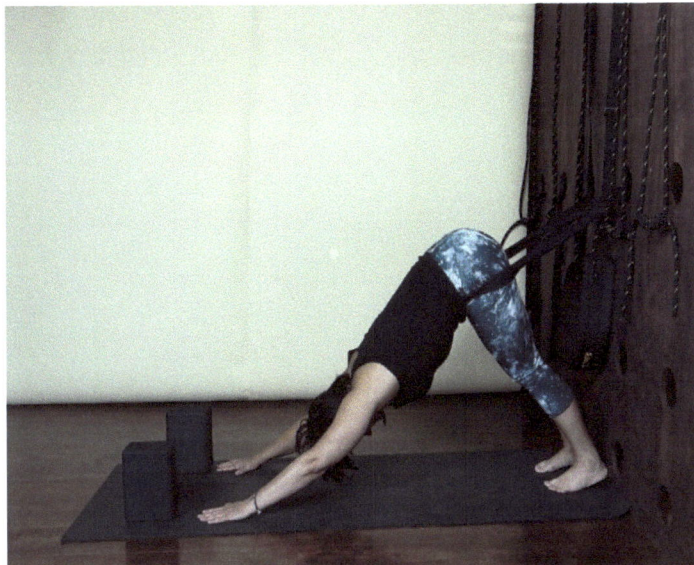

Another variation is to add a twist, drawing the hand across to the opposite calf or ankle.

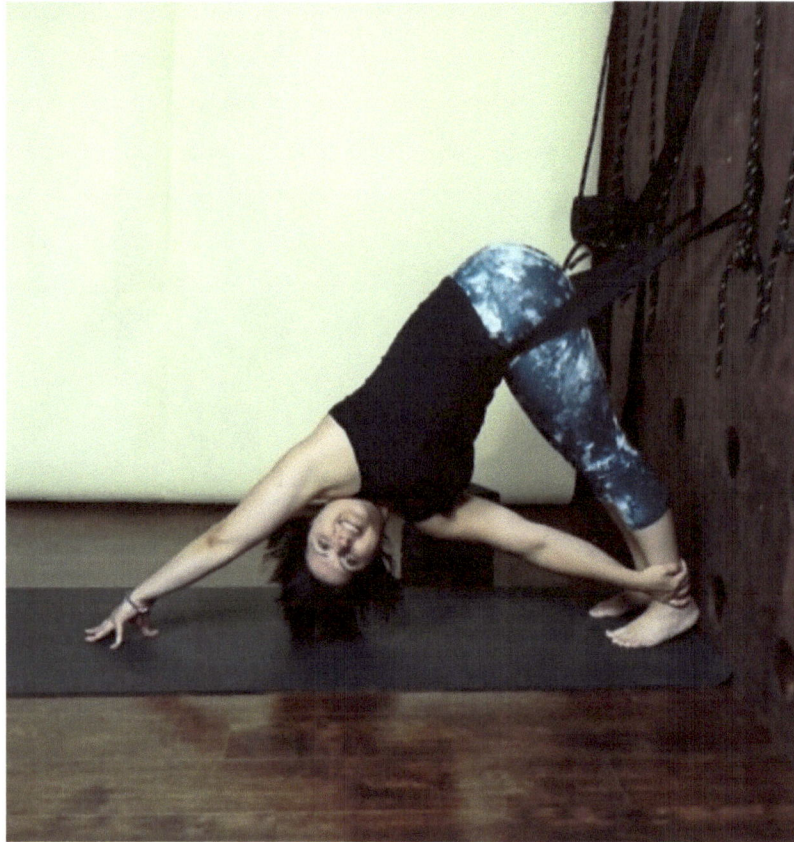

Pyramid Pose

Lift up from Down Dog and put your hands back on the blocks. Walk the blocks in so that they are under your shoulders. Lift the chest, then step one leg forward as far as you can without shifting in the rope, finding Pyramid Pose.

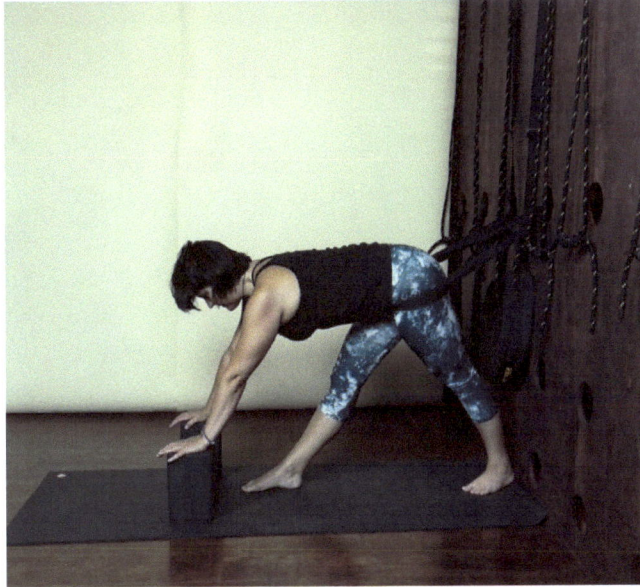

Notice what happens if I try to put my hands on the floor. Notice how my back is rounded.

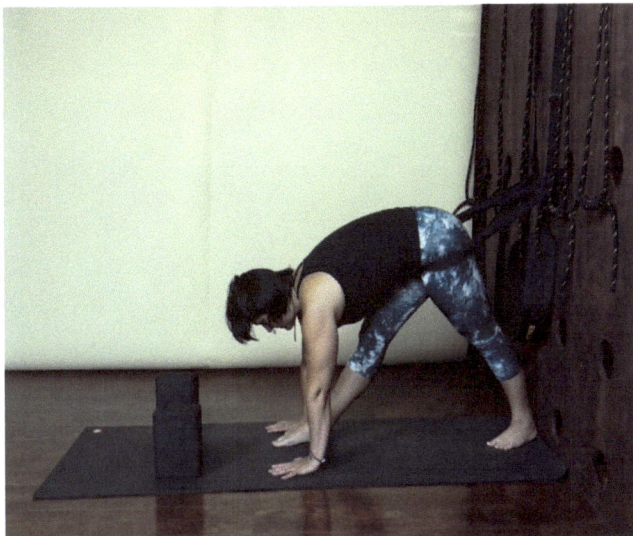

Revolved Pyramid

From pyramid pose, lift up and twist around, grabbing for the high rope farthest behind you. Hold it high and slide down until your hand comes back to the block. This is your revolved pyramid. Work to open the chest to the opposite side.

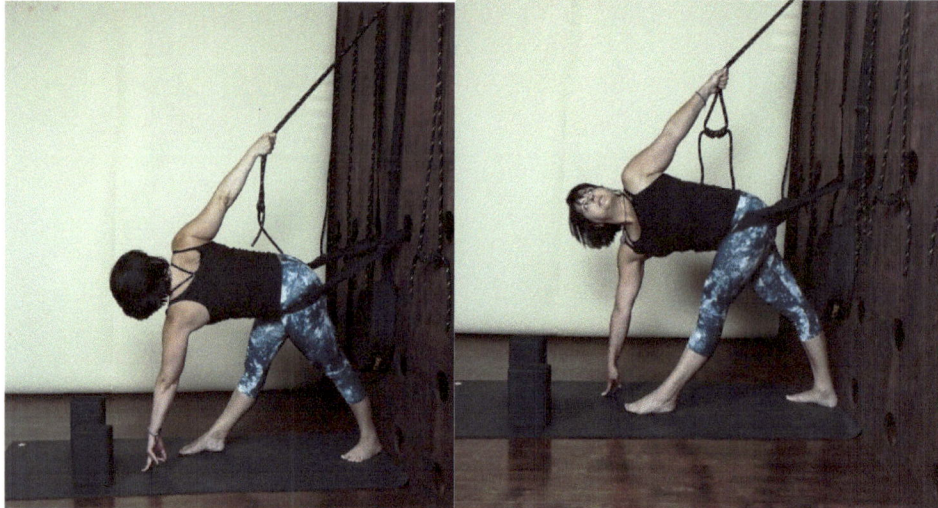

Come back to Downward Dog then work through the other side. It is fun to to work with Triangle Pose in the low ropes, as well. I do not have photos, but keep the ropes where they are above and open up to the side to slide out into triangle.

Low Low Ropes and Pilates Exercises

Bringing the ropes down to the knee level handles offers a few nice exercises, including a series of Pilates based exercises. There are more Pilates exercises in the Knee High Sling section.

Lunges

It is helpful to learn to draw the hips in line in our lunges and this variation helps us to find that. Place the rope around the leg that will be drawn back. Come down into the tension and drop the knee down. Place the hands on the wall and work the leg back as far as you can, allowing the rope to hold the hip in place. The higher you lift the chest the more you will feel the stretch of the psoas. Pushing into the wall with the hands may help.

If you'd like to move on, lift the back knee off the floor and come to a more traditional lunge. Make sure your front knee is not reaching forward. If this is a problem, you might put a block between the knee and the wall and work to hold it in place.

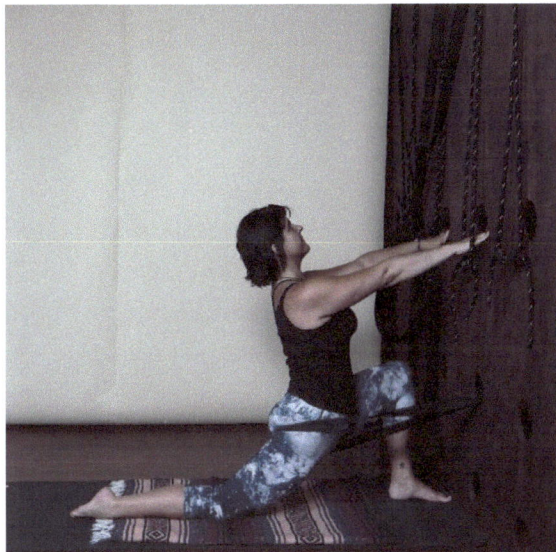

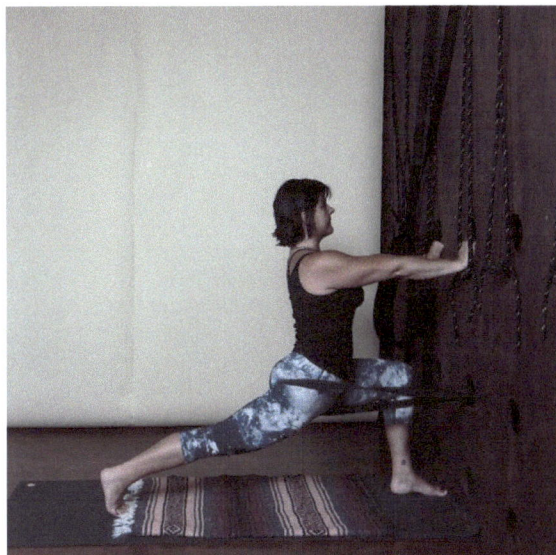

Lizard

In a similar vein, working with lizard in this way can be helpful. Bring the loop onto the inner thigh all the way up to the crease. Make sure there is tension and come down into your lizard. Notice how resisting the tension helps to get deeper into the hip.

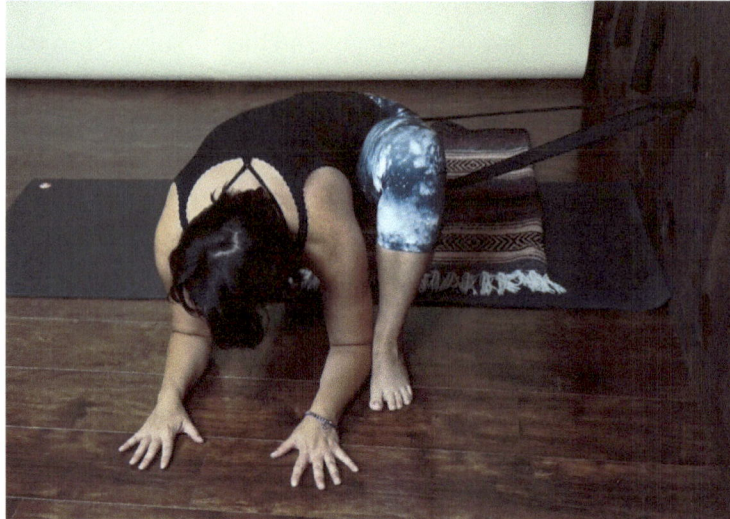

The tension and need to pull against it allows more understanding of drawing the hip closer. It also distracts the proprioceptors and creates confusion so the muscles let go and the stretch becomes deeper.

Here are a few more variations to use the low ropes in traditional poses.

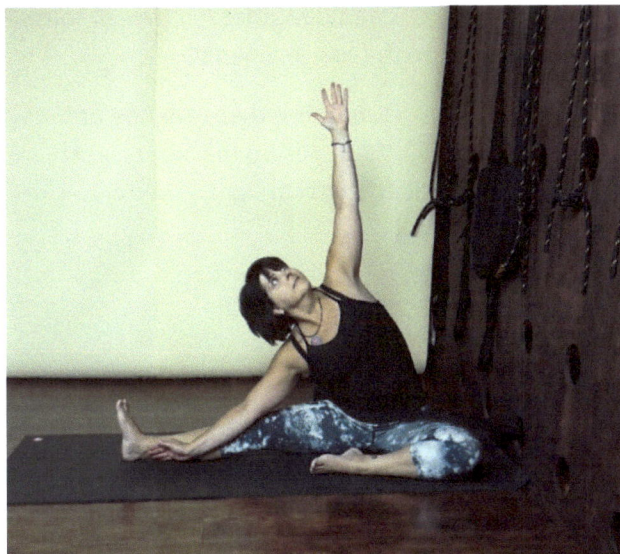

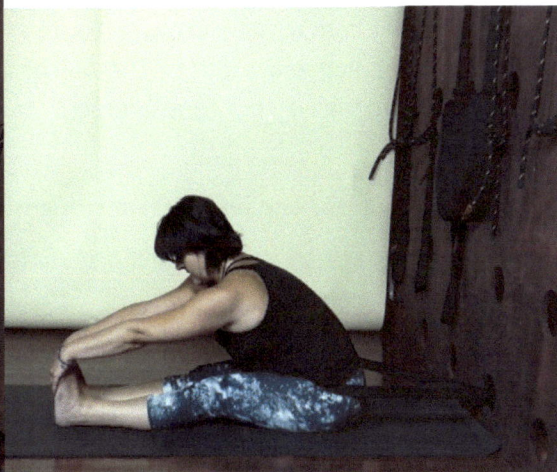

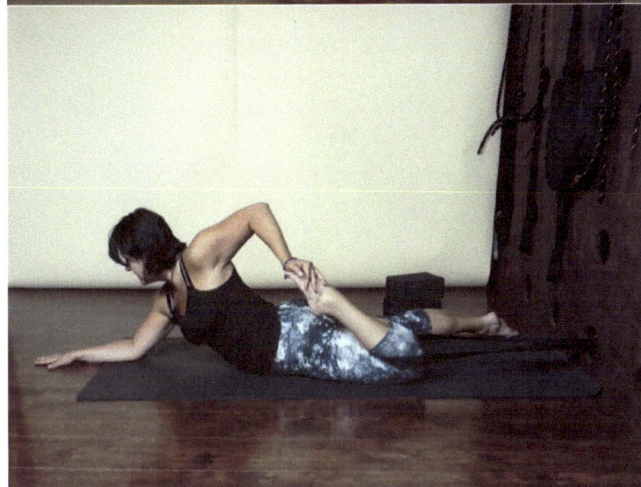

Pilates Exercises

I noticed while arranging these pictures that the ropes are on the high handle for these, however some of them, such as happy baby and the hip stretches might be better on the low low handle.

Begin with the feet both in the low ropes. For the first exercises it won't matter if there are one or two ropes on both feet. Put your hands on the wall or the low handles. Put the ropes on the ankles. Push yourself away from the wall but keep your legs straight. If you can't keep them straight, move closer to the wall.

Sink down into your hips and feel the hamstring stretch.

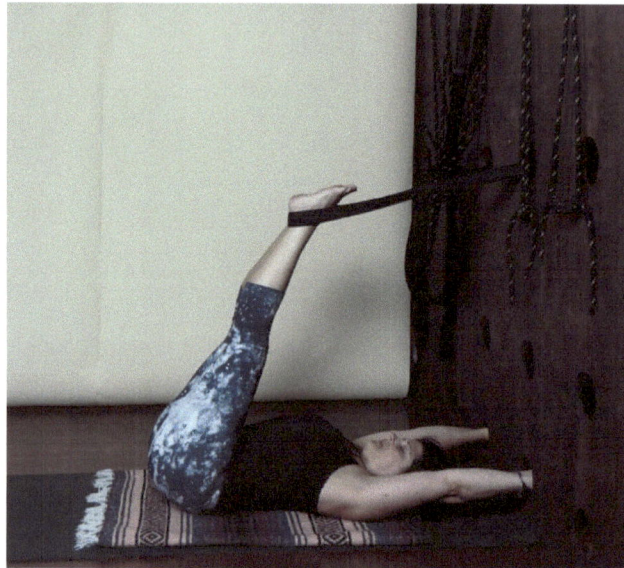

When you are ready, lift up through the legs and press the feet towards the ceiling.

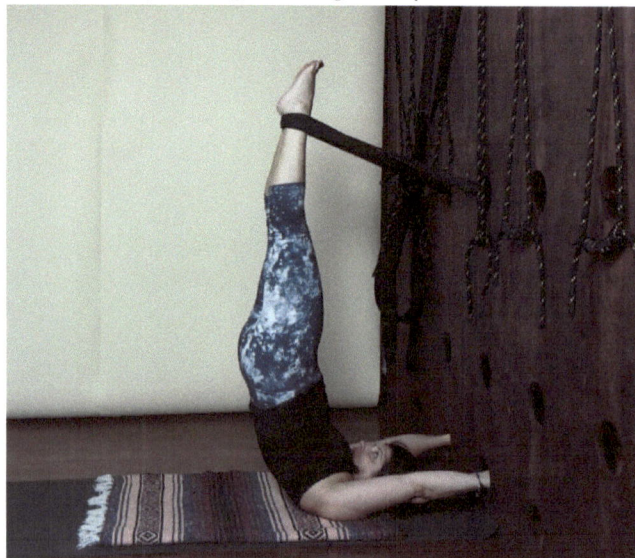

After 8-10 rounds, release one foot from the ropes, and lower it down and away, hovering it off the floor.

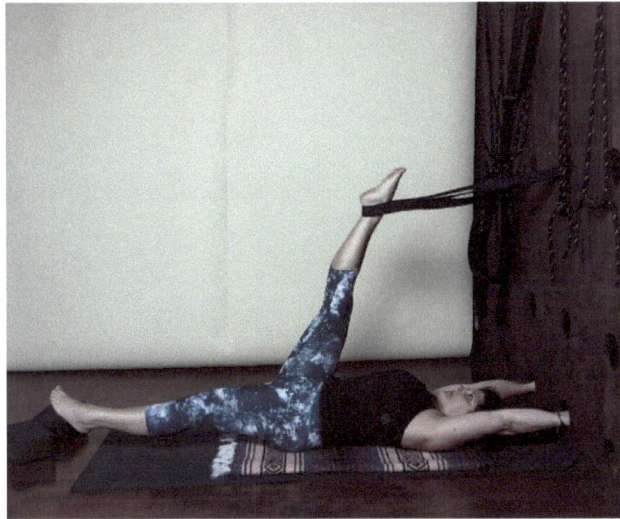

Then lift up into that one leg, drawing the other leg up to meet it. Make sure to stay long in both legs throughout this exercise, feeling the deeper hamsring stretch on the way down.

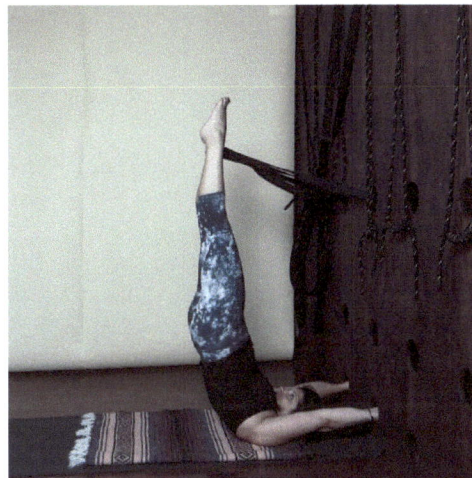

The next few stretches would be great on the low low handles.

Happy Baby

Complete 8-10 rounds on each side then Put both legs into separate ropes and find a happy baby.

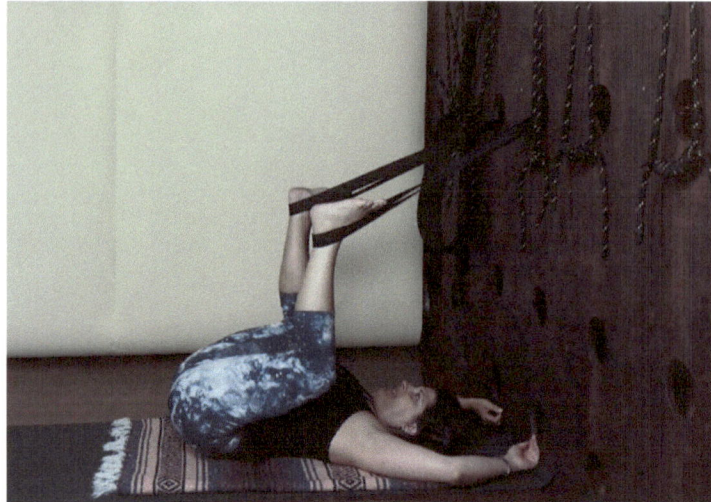

Hamstring and Hip Stretches.

Remove one foot from the loop and come into a hamstring stretch. Allow the other leg to drop completely.

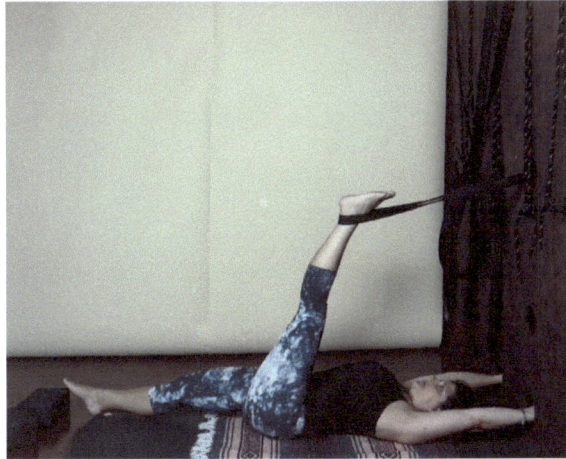

Allow that leg to stay straight and draw it open, turning the toes slightly down.

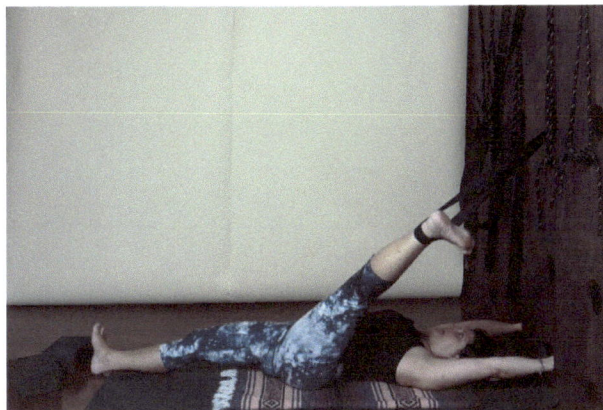

Place the foot ino the opposite look and allow the foot to be drw across the body, first with a straight leg, then a bent knee.

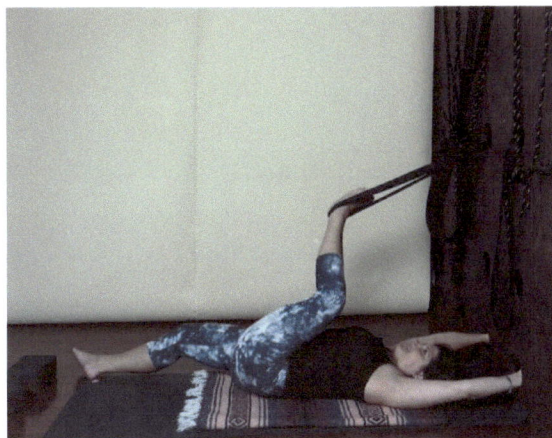

Pilates Advance Control

As a final exercise in this series, put each leg in separate ropes and lift up.

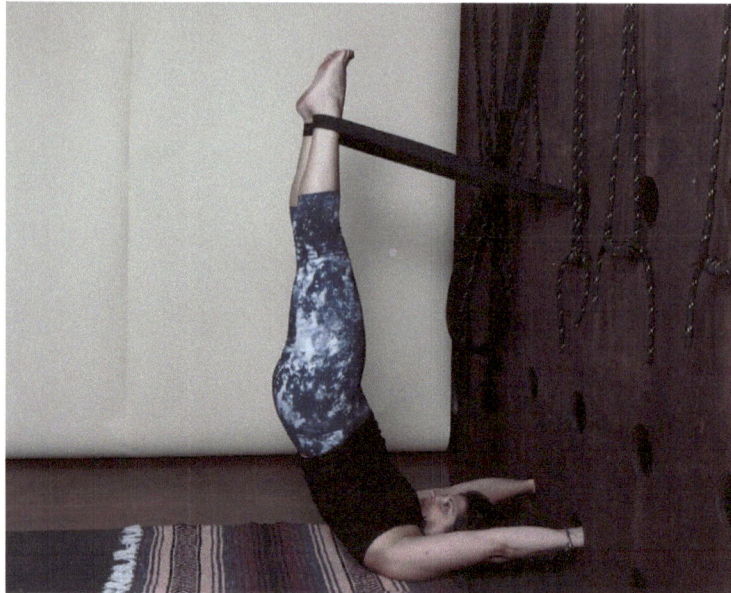

While your legs are up, open them, then close them and lower back down. Repeat 8-10 times.

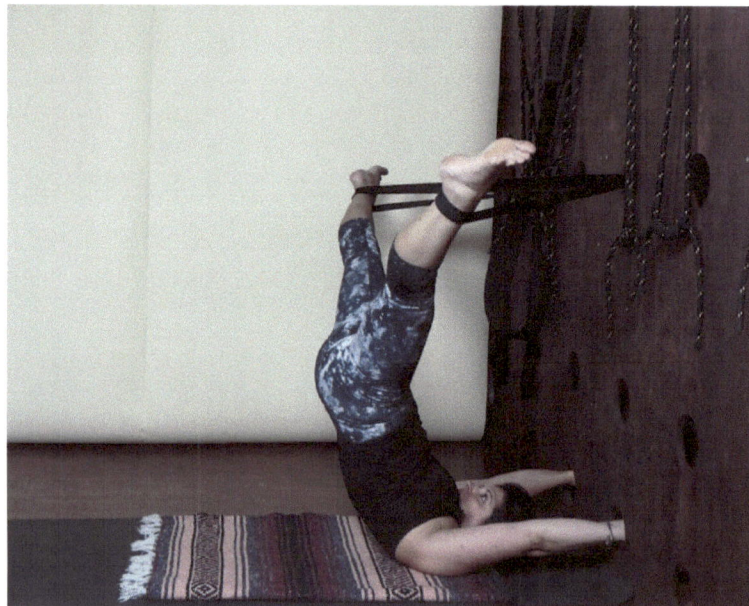

Low Handles and Seated Work

While there are a lot of things that can be done with the low handles, this book will only offer a few. If you do not have handles on your wall, using a chair or other piece of furniture may work for most of these.

Seated Forward Fold

Begin seated with feet on the wall. Those who are less flexible can hold the high ropes, pulling down in the arms as they draw their chest up and towards the wall.

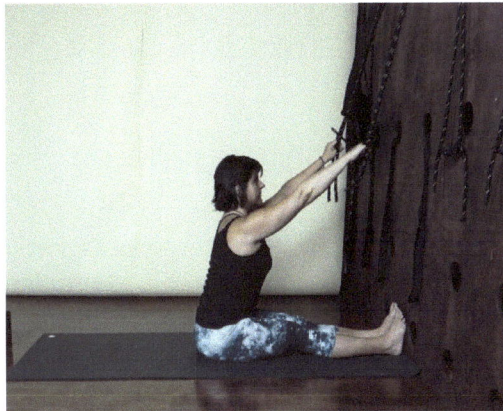

The next step would be to walk your hands down and grab the knee height handles. Gently walk your sits bones back as you offer your heart forward. Finally, if available to you, walk the hands down to hold the lower handles, maintaining the hips back.

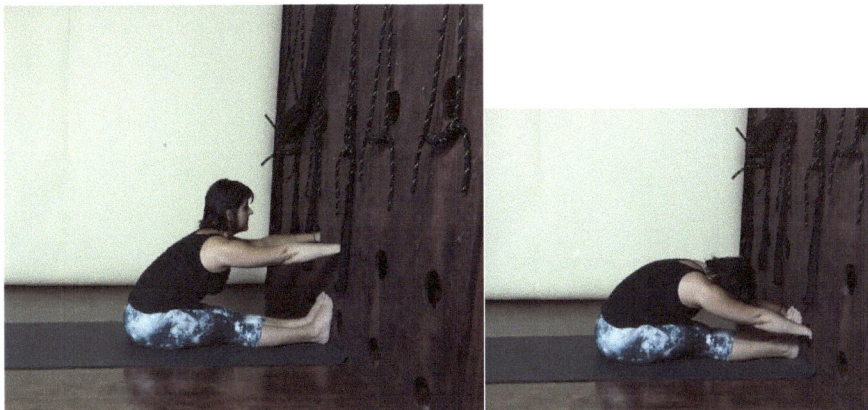

Variations of Janu shirasana can also be done here.

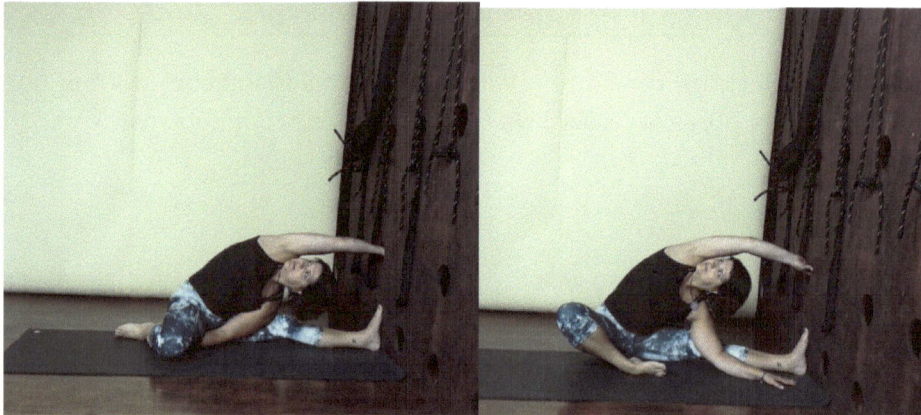

Seated Twist

Holding the high ropes. Sit facing the wall, feet against it and holding the high ropes. Open the free arm out to the side taking the chest along.

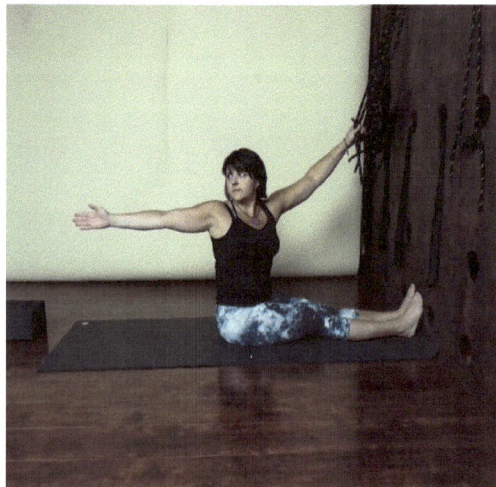

Boat Pose Variation

Sit facing the wall. Hold the high ropes and bring your feet up on the wall. Work to lift the chest.

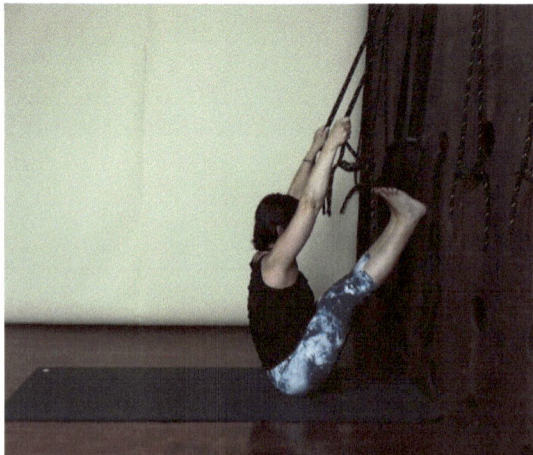

Straddle

Simply sit facing the wall with feet open. Gently pull yourself to the wall, pushing through the heels until you get to the point of discomfort. Push through the heels and keep lifting the chest. It may be possible to pull a little farther after a few breaths, but always use caution.

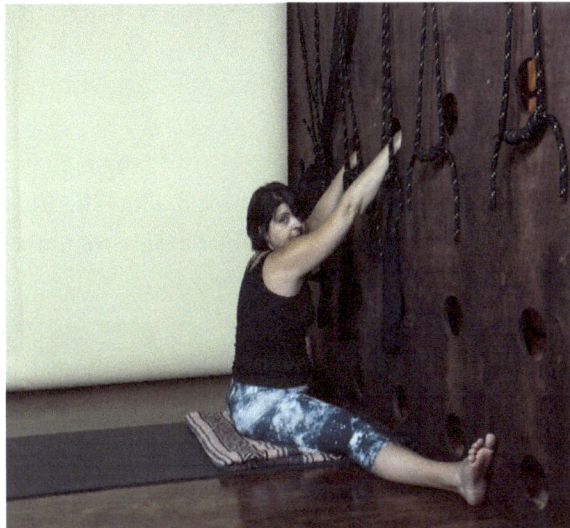

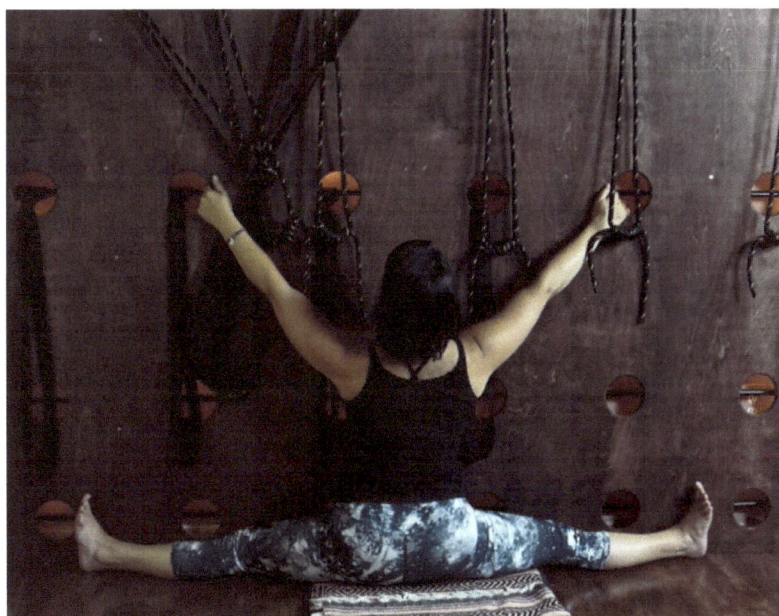

High Handles

This a good place to work on shoulder openings or warrior 3 to get the hips I alignment. The same could be done with a chair or even with hands on the wall.

I offer a few other poses here to help deepen hip openers and a backbend.

Camel

Stand on your knees with hips and knees touching the wall. Hold the high handles. Lift up through the lower back and chest. Keep the hips and knees at the wall and allow the upper back to lift up and arch back. If you have a neck issue, do not allow the head to fall back; work more from the upper back and keep the chin forward. To come out, simply lift the head and sit back.

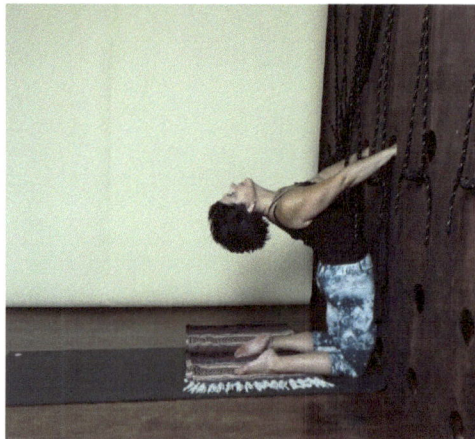

For another variation of this pose, stand on your knees with your toes on the wall facing away. Lifting from the hips, press them forward and reach your hands back to the wall. If you can reach in and grab the handles, then hold them as you work your hips farther forward and your chest up.

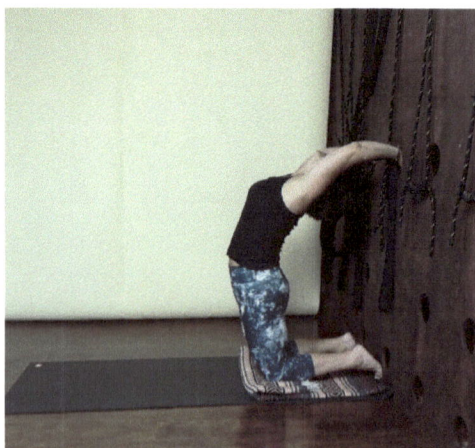

Similarly, one can work towards their toe grips in this way. Come to a lunge or pigeon legs, with the knee to the wall and foot lifted (shin on the wall). Sink down into the hips and work the arms back to grab the handles. Work to puff your chest forward while pulling on the handles. Please use caution in this variation as it is a deep back bend and shoulder opener.

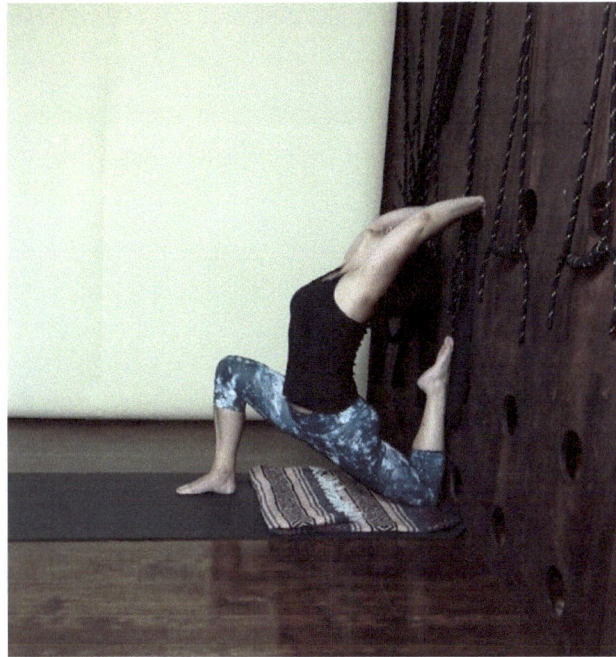

Another variation is a hanumanasana reach back. The directions are the same as he last pose, however with the front leg straight.

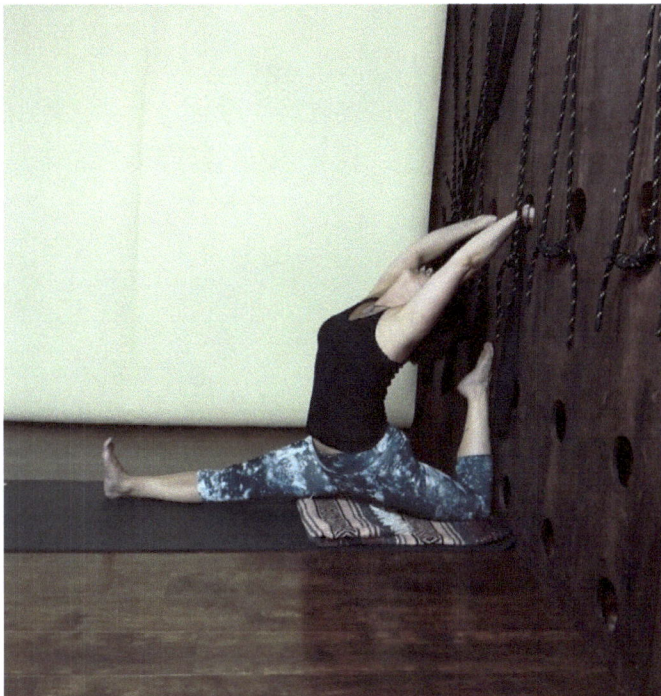

SLINGS

Ah, the sling. This is usually everyone's favorite part of working on the wall. There are many different exercises that can be done on the sling so I have broken them down by height of the sling. Most slings are adjustable, however it can be cumbersome to go back and forth between heights so I suggest grouping exercises together according to the height to be used.

There are three main heights. Knee (mid- level) height, hip (highest) height and ankle (lowest) height. They generally work in that manner, however adjustments may need to be made for comfort and ease of movement.

Please remember: when working with slings they should be used on the pelvic bones – not the soft part of the stomach or on the spine. Some backbends do utilize the lower back position, but doing so properly and with caution is imperative.

Sling Knee Height

To begin, lower the sling to knee height (when hanging straight down it lands about mid-knee). Make sure you have two blocks or a chair in front of you so that you have something to reach for to begin. Stand with your back to the wall and the sling in front of you. Walk out until the sling is at your hips and lean weight into it. Bend down to place your hands on blocks or the chair, then walk your feet back to the wall, keeping weight in the sling.

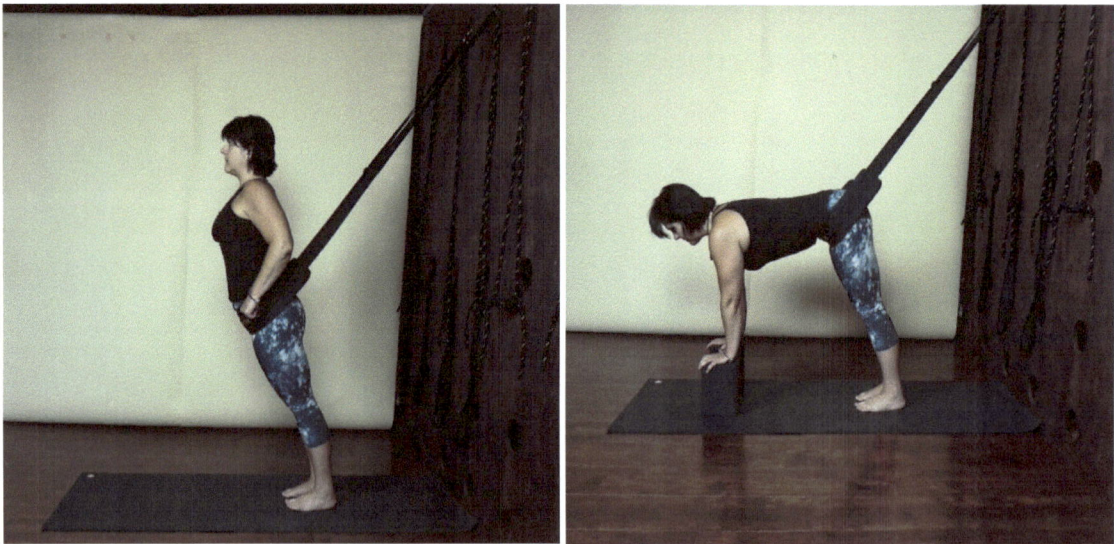

Once your feet are at the wall, you can lift the heels and stay on the balls of the toes. Make sure your heels remain connected to the wall. Walk the hands on the blocks out and away until your arms are extended. If you are able to maitain strenth in the shoulders and a long spine, you can allow your hands to come to the floor. You may evenbe able to allow the elbows to come down, as in Dolphin.

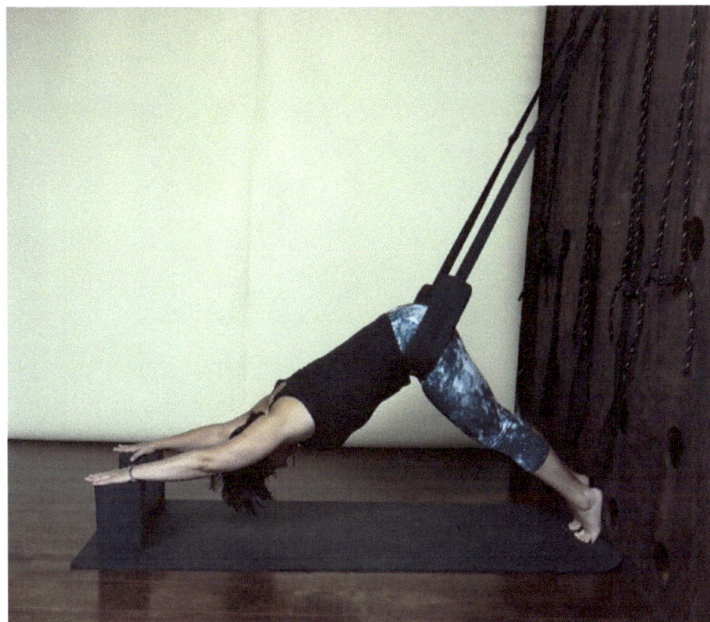

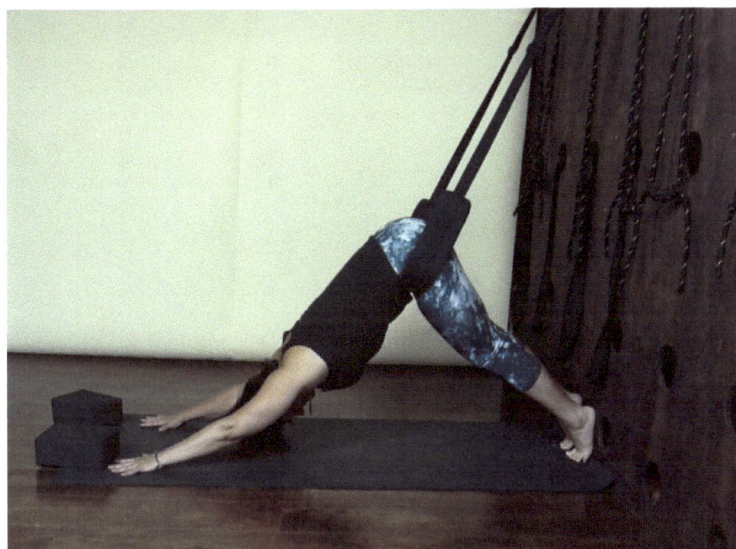

It's nice to sway the hips from side to side here, allowing some movement in the lower spine and pelvis. Remain here for a while.

Back Extensions

When you are ready to move on, Bend the knees and squat back, still hanging in the sling.

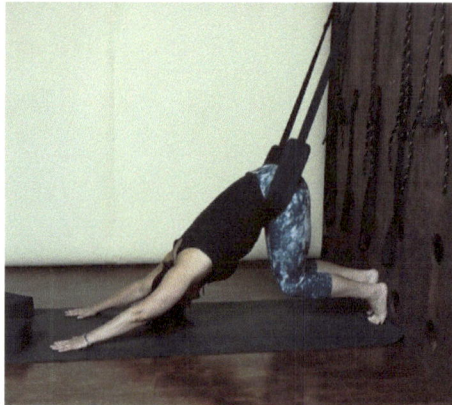

Press out from the feet and straighten the legs. See if you can allow your fingertips to dangle off the floor. This is your prep test for the back extension series. If you feel any pain in the back then it is best not to move on and to consult a doctor.

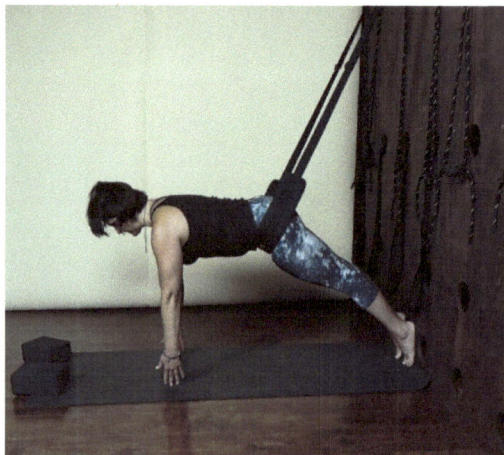

Now, go back to your squatted legs, then alternate the squat with the reach out as you move through the exercise. Arm position may vary. If you have back tension it may be best to leave the hands along the sides like airplane wings (think masthead of a ship).

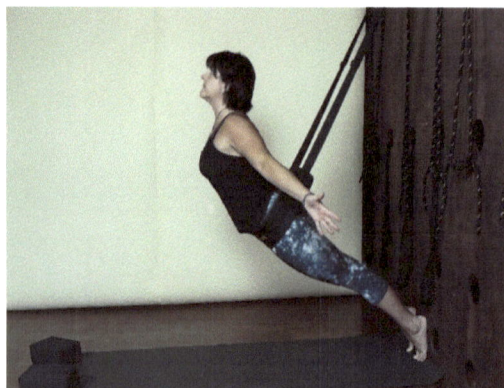

Otherwise, bring the hands up in front of you like superman. This variation is more strain on the low back, so use caution.

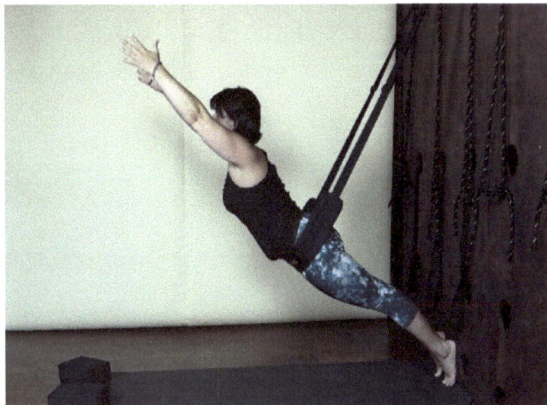

Another variation is to Twist open to one side and lift. This will work each side separately.

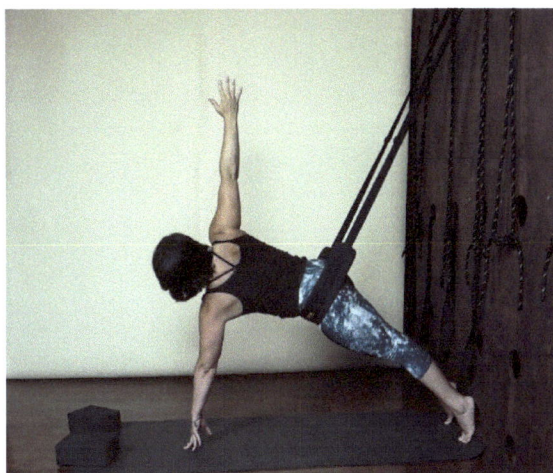

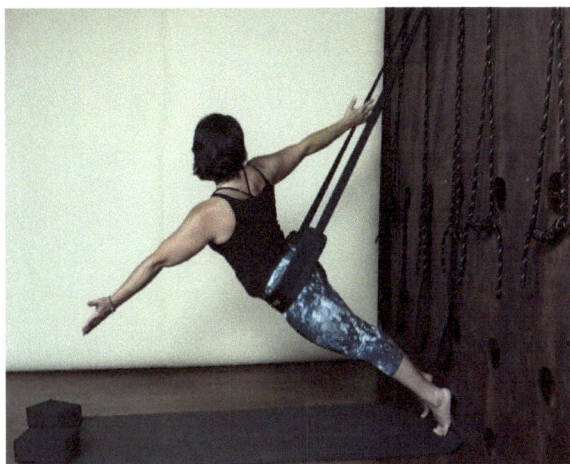

Supported Side Plank Variation

This may look similar to the last exercise, however, you will notice the hips have been turned in the sling to face the side. This exercise can also be done with the sling at the rib cage, possibly needing to adjust the length of the sling to make it slightly longer. Both variations are quite nice and should be tried. Place the foot from the top leg in front of the bottom one.

After you have gotten into position, see if you can lift up. This is a great exercise for the waist and mid back. Also, you can place a block under the hand or lower the sling to make this more supportive.

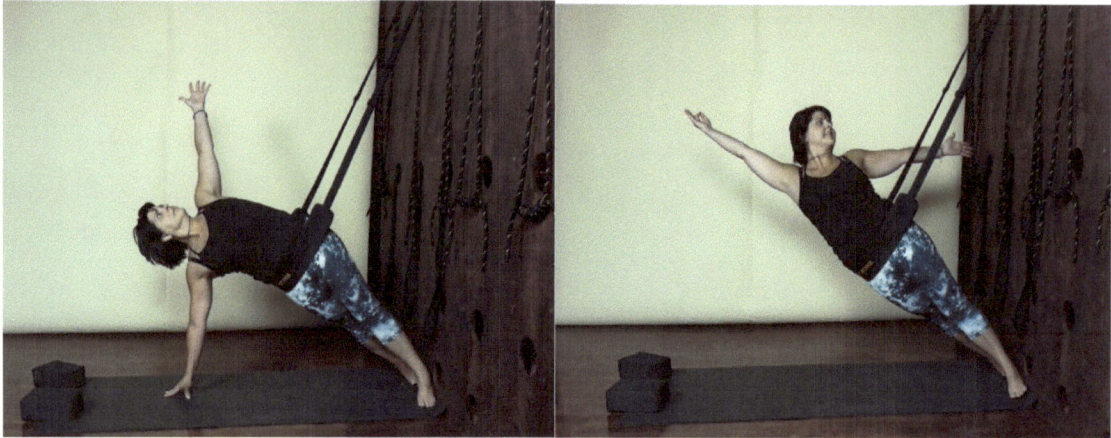

After you do the exercise, this is a nice time to stretch the arm over the head into a side bend. The lower knee may need to bend.

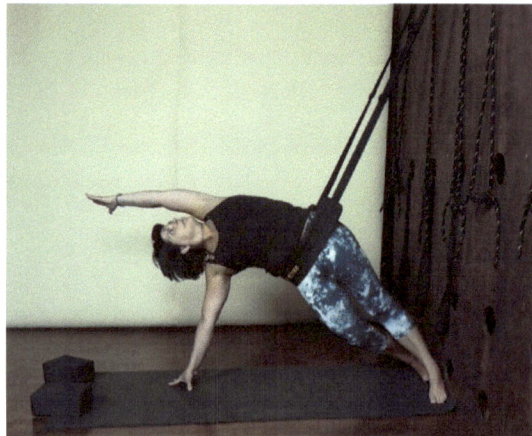

Wild Thing

From Side plank, Wild thing can be nice for some practitioners, although please use caution with shoulders. You have to have the sling at the hips for this one.

Simply begin to walk your top foot up the wall and over to the opposite side, as high as you can. Allow your top arm and chest to fall back, supported. This is a lovely, supported back and chest stretch.

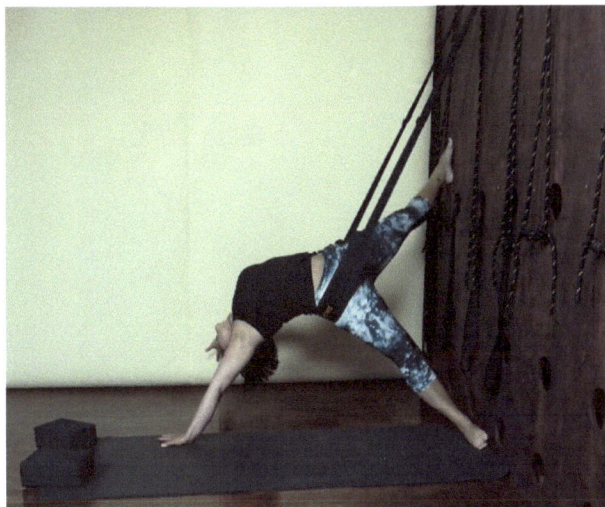

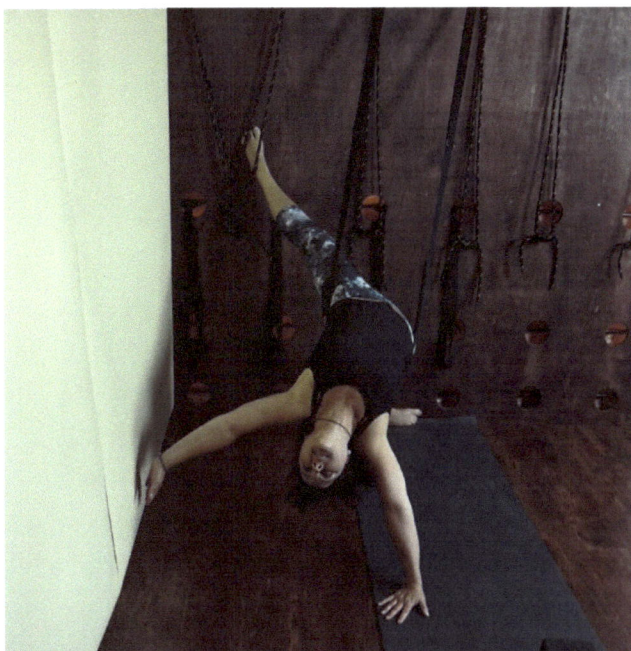

And now a fan favorite.

Child's Pose

Keeping the weight in the sling, simply place one knee, then the other onto the wall and allow the knees to drop as low as they can as you bring your forehead to the floor and extend the arms.

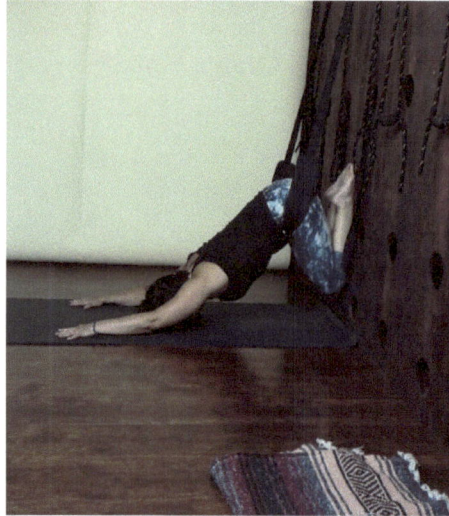

It's nice to try a twisted variation here, as well. Just draw one arm and shoulder under the other and across to the other side of the mat. Walk the other hand up and over the head, if desired. Draw the ear to the mat.

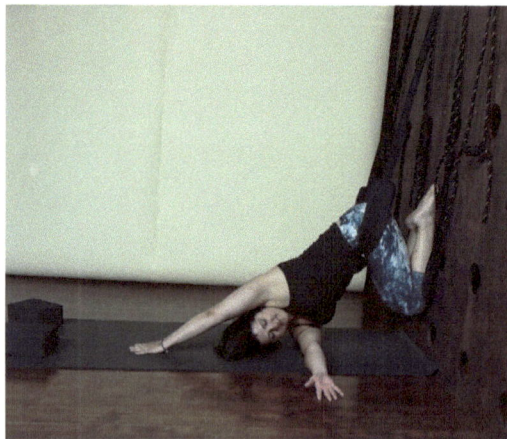

***This pose can also be done in a more inverted format with the sling raised to the high level. It is a wonderful inversion and you can add some shoulder stretches. It's a great alternative to hanging backwards for those who that may not be appropriate for.

Pilates Bridge Lifts

Another Pilates series that can be done is with the sling at knee height.

Lie on your back, feet towards the wall with ankles in the sling and legs extended. Mae sure your feet don't quite touch the wall when the legs are fully extended. This alone can bring some nice relief to back pain, but another nice choice is to "fishtail" the legs, swinging them side to side. This can be done for a nice relaxation, even by those who want a gentle practice.

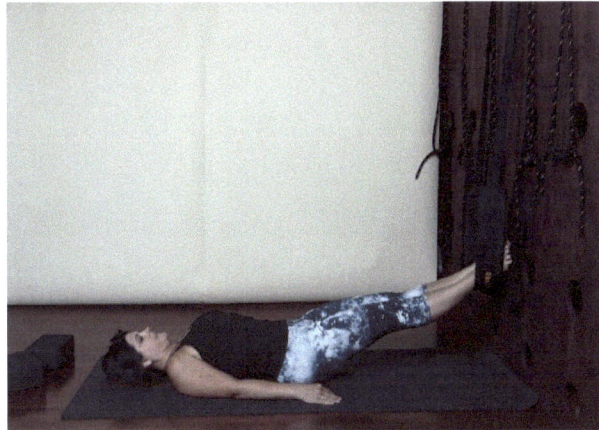

This exercise is a powerful hamstring workout. With legs in sling, press into the heels and lift the bottom off the floor.

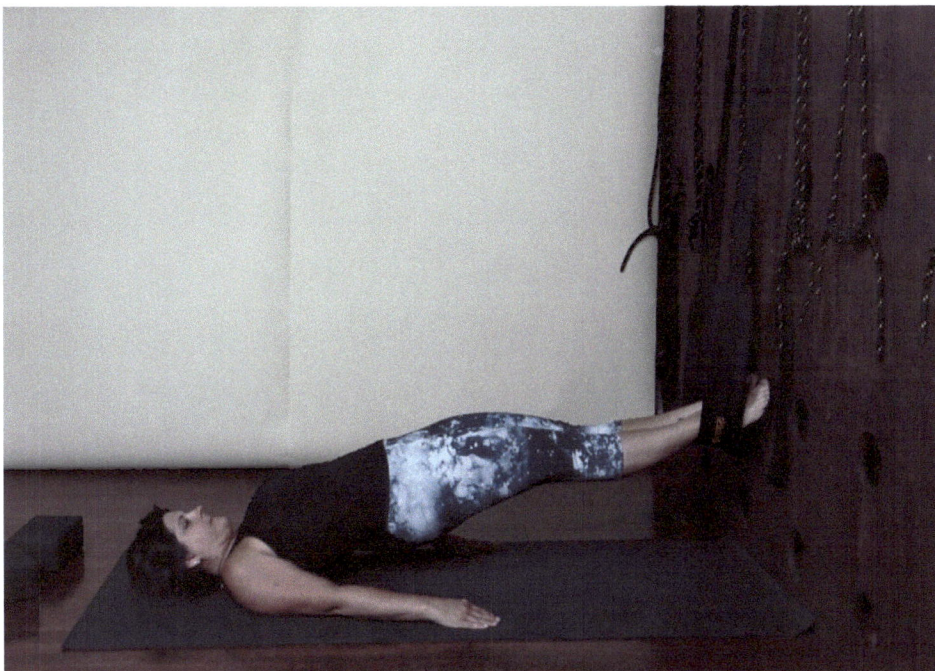

Keeping the botom up, draw the feet towards you into a bridge position. Hold up, then press the feet back out and lower down. Make sure to keep the core strong to support the back.

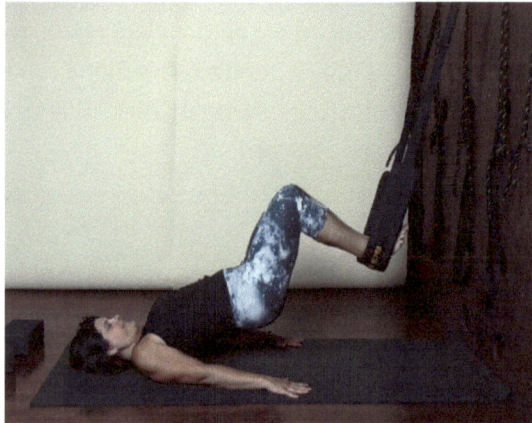

This exercise can be tried with the legs turned out in Plie, ot lifting one foot off the floor.

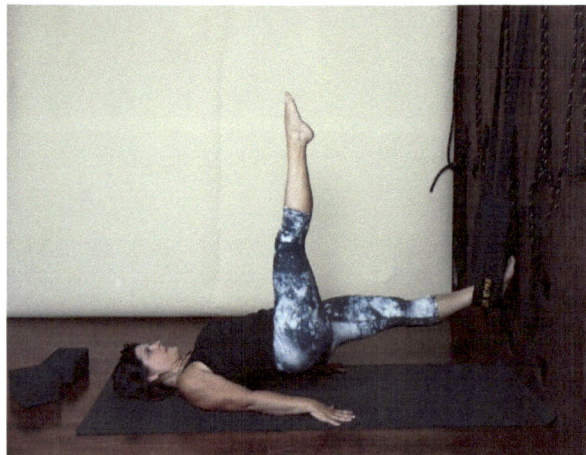

For a welcome rest, move closer to the wall, draw the sling to the knees and rest.

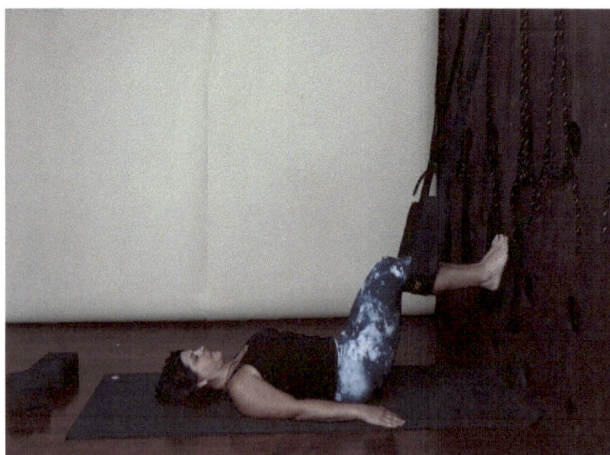

Wheel Pose

If you are working on wheel pose, this is one variaton that will assist you. This one is done at the knee height.

Facing the wall with the sling at your hips behind you, put your feet at the wall and press your knees into it. Hold the sling as you lower back, allowing your hips to be suported by the sling. This may be all you do for a while, until you feel ready to progress. You could allow your head to rest on a block, if desired.

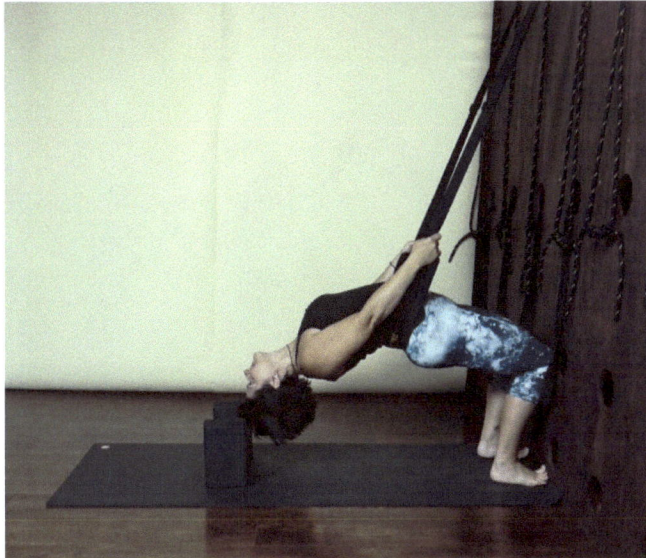

Next, let go of the sling and bring the hands to blocks, or possibly the floor.

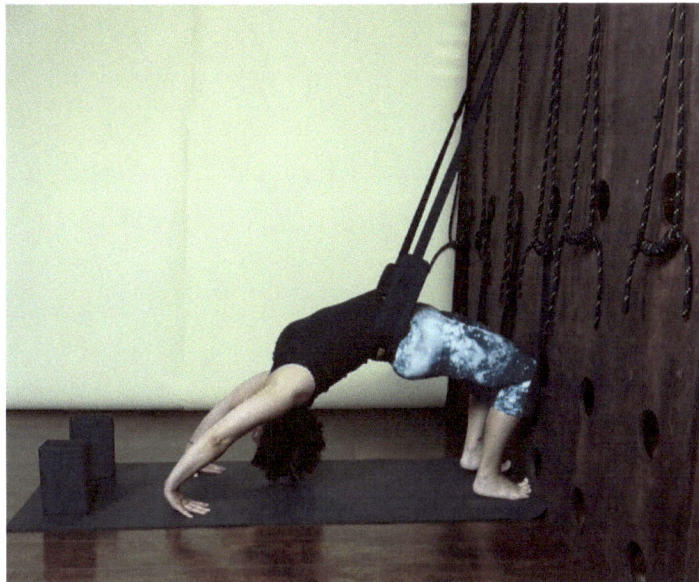

Finally, if all else is well, straighten the legs. This is a deep backbend and should only be worked up to.

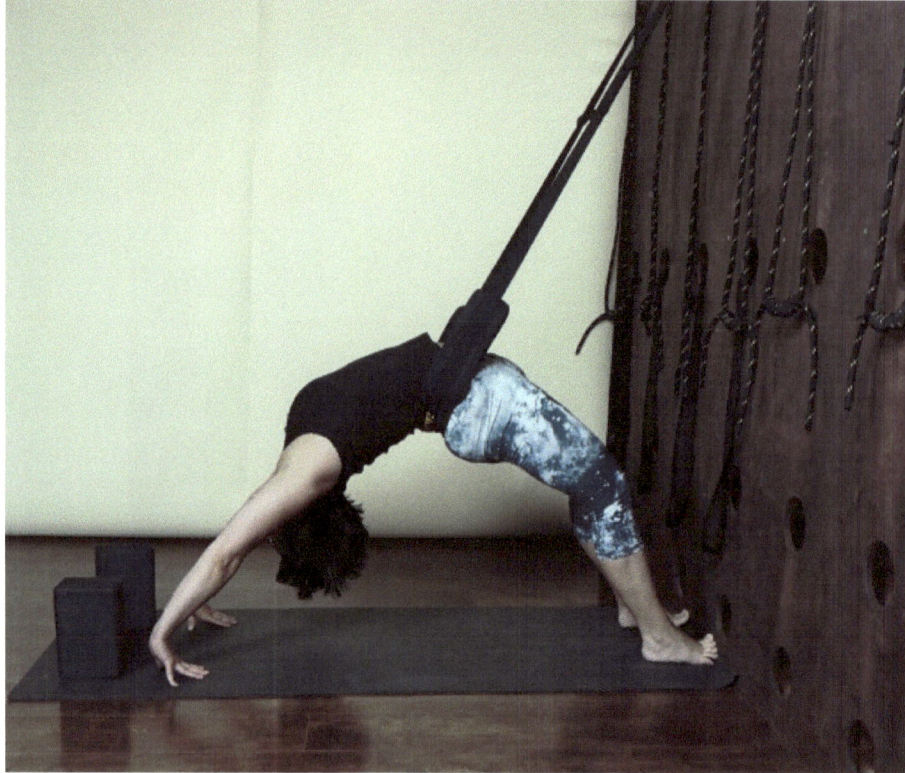

Table Top Hip Stretches

Coming onto the knees and hands or forearms, place one foot into the sling. Turn the knee down and lean back into the legs.The sling leg will be drawn back and into a deep hip flexor opener.

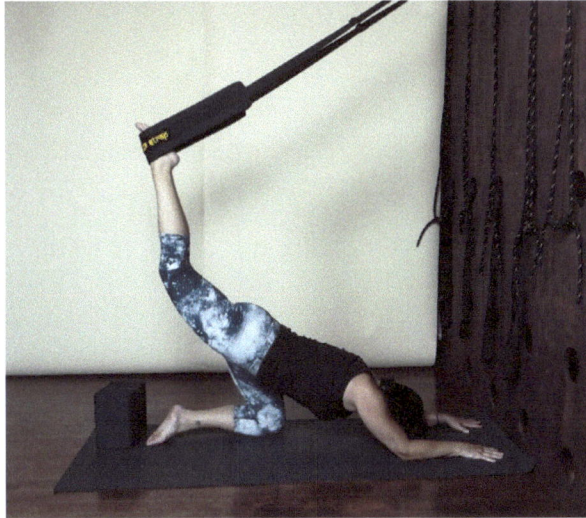

Draw the sling foot out to the side for an inner thigh stretch. It will be helpful to come up onlo the hands and you may even be able to slide sideways, to a degree, to get deeper.

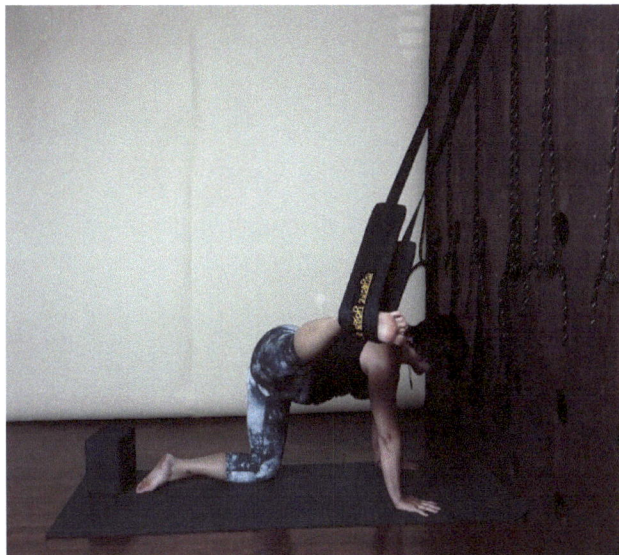

These can also be done from down dog, as you will see later in the high slings chapter.

These next few poses may need the sling brought up a litle, but not all the way up. Please adjust as necessary.

Warrior 3

Face away from the wall and bring the sling to your hipbones, leaning into it. Make sure you are far enough away and lift your back foot to the wall. Fold down and bring your hands to the floor or blocks. Lift the foot back and place it on the wall.

The foot should be roughly at hip height (these photos show the foot a little higher). Press into the toes and engage the foot.

Lift the arms up and forward, or along the sides like airplane wings. Think about the length in the spine.

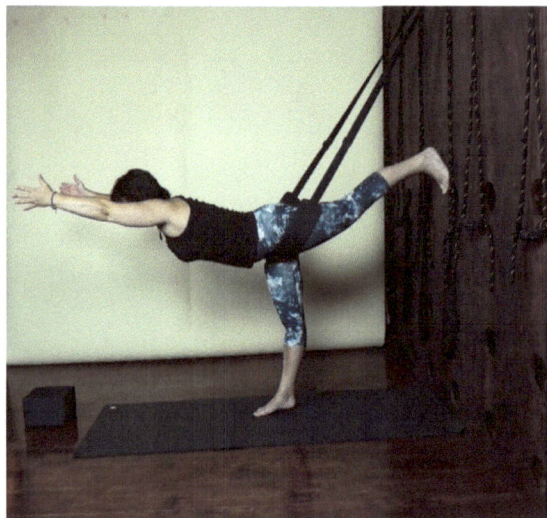

Twisted variation. From Warrior 3, place hands back on the floor and work to open the opposite hand of the wall leg up, twisting the chest open towards the standin leg side of the room. Beginners should put the hand on the hip before attempting to reach up.

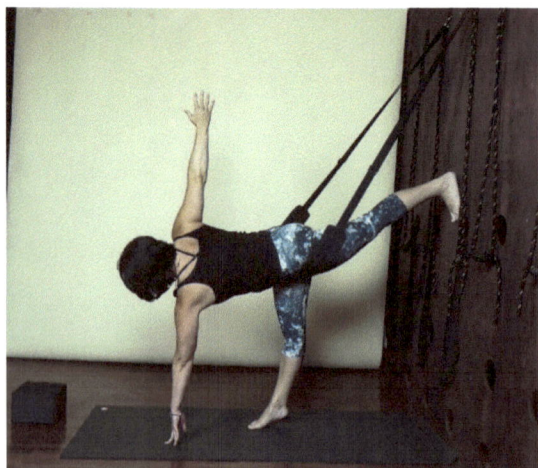

Standing Split

From the warrior variations, draw the hands back to the floor and lean into the sling. Lift the wall leg off the wall and up behind you, as far as possible. Keep the weight in the sling. Draw the head down towards the shin of the standing leg. This pose on the wall eliminates some of the balance so you can experience a deeper variation. Note that the back foot does not require contact with the wall.

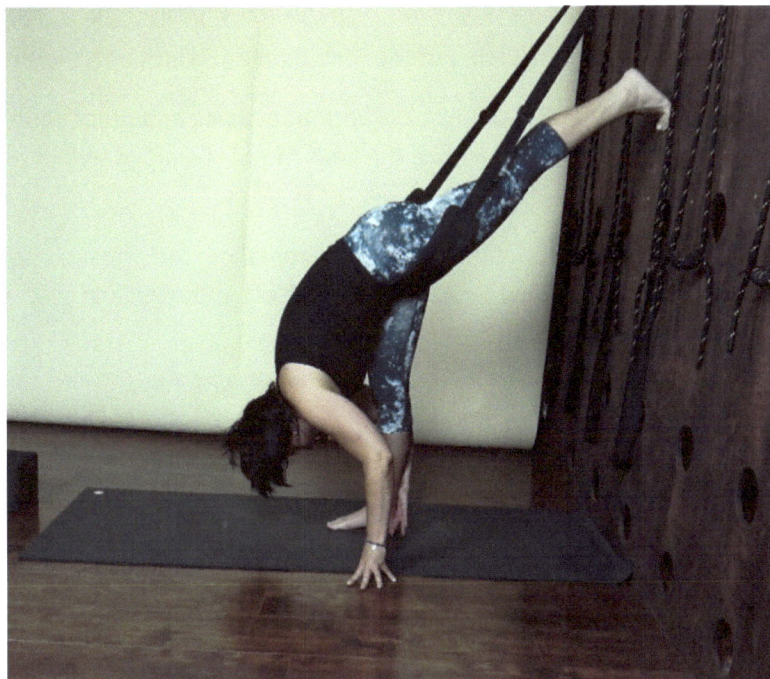

Sling High Height

Bring the sling up to the highest level for these poses. Shorter bodies may need it slightly lower.

Lay Backs

Face the wall and put the sling under your shoulder blades/armpits. Walk back and put weight into the sling and then walk your feet back to the wall. Put the feet shoulder width apart with a slight turn out.

Begin with the hands behind the head to support. Lay your head back and press your head into your hands. Resist the pressure with your hands. Notice the back muscles start to work. It's nice to also sway side to side here.

Now, if you do not have any neck issues, let go of the head and allow the arms to open to the sides. It can be nice to "backstroke" the arms a few times. Once you feel supported and safe, allow the upper body to lay back and hang, supported by the sling.

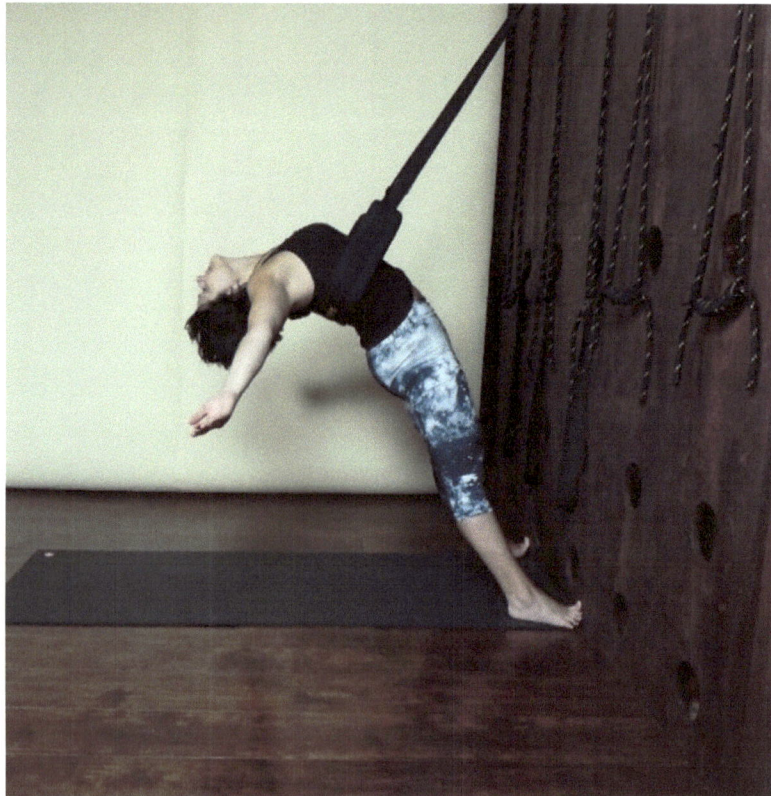

It is also nice here to bend one knee and lean towards that side, swinging side to side with a stretch. Bring the arm overhead and windmill he hands for a nice dance (not shown).

Prayer Squat Hang

This is a nice resting position and, consequently, is WONDERFUL for pregnant women and those with lower back tenderness.

From the layback position, gently bend the knees and drop the hips, coming to a squat at the wall. Reach the hands up or simply allow them to hang. It is also nice to do some pelvic tilts and releases in this position as the lower back will have some space to move.

Come out by extending the legs, keeping weight in the sling, and walking back.

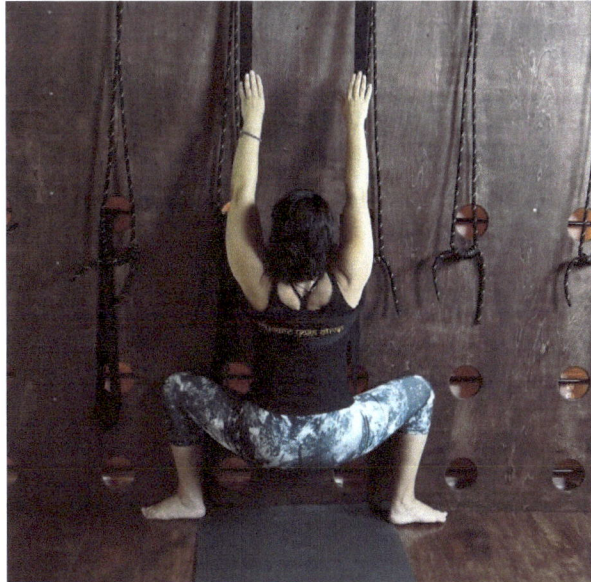

Side Lunge – Extended Side Angle with Support

Backing out of the prayer squat, extend one leg, reaching towards the opposite side. It may be possible to grab hold of a handle here. Lift the toes of the extended leg. Keen the bent knee at the wall for support.

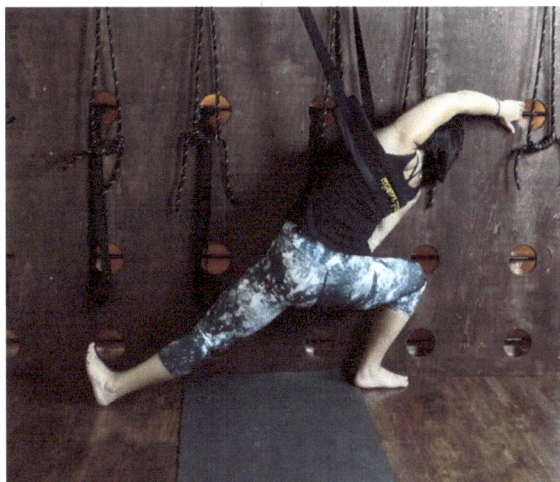

Hanging - Baddha Konasana

This is undoubtedly one of the favorites.

Please make sure the *sling is high enough that your head will clear the floor when you go back*. For most people, this will be the highest setting, however, very short people or kids may find this somewhat difficult to get into.

To get in, stand facing the wall and bring the sling behind you to the hips. Walk out and put tension into the sling.

Hold the straps of the sling as you walk your feet up the wall – like a mountain climber. **KEEP THE KNEES AND FEET WIDE**. When your feet are about the height of the sling, squat down to the wall – **OPENING THE KNEES OUTSIDE OF THE STRAPS**. Keep looking at your navel.

Walk the hands down the straps, keeping the legs wide and the face looking at the navel. Before releasing the hands, wrap your feet in front of the straps. Continue releasing one hand at a time to the floor until you know you have support.

Tuck your bottom and try to bring the length of the spine to the wall.

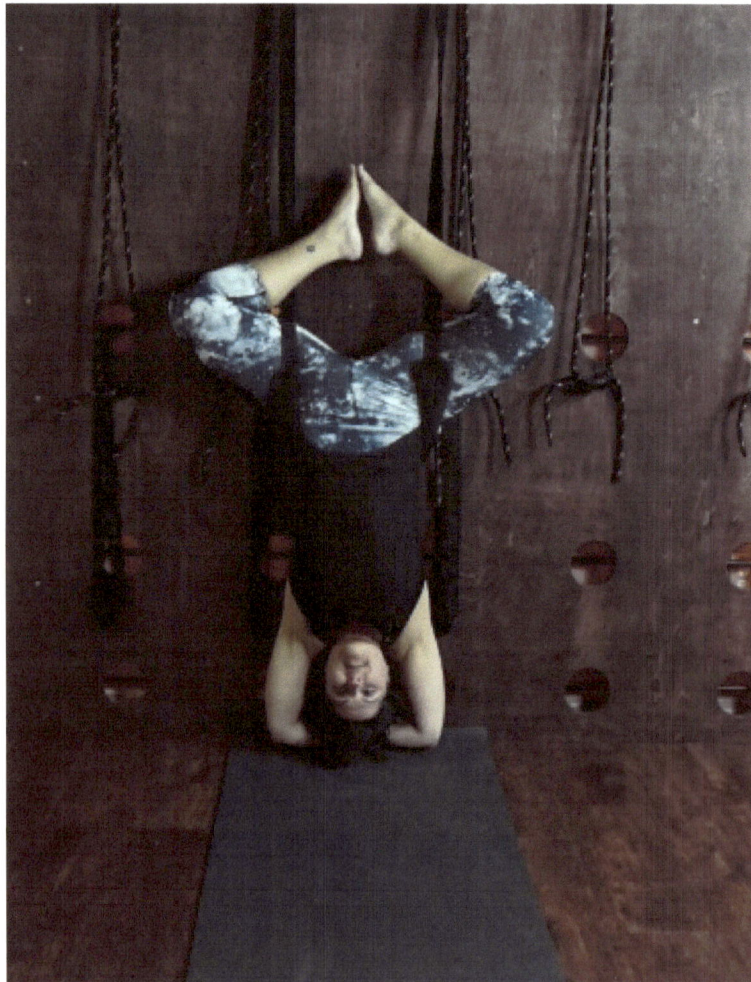

To come out, look up at your navel. Reach up and grab the straps. Walk up as high as you can and unravel the legs – but keep them wide (this is a safety feature). I like to do a little forward bend here by walking my hands up as high as I can while lifting up my torso. Please keep the legs wrapped under the straps, though.

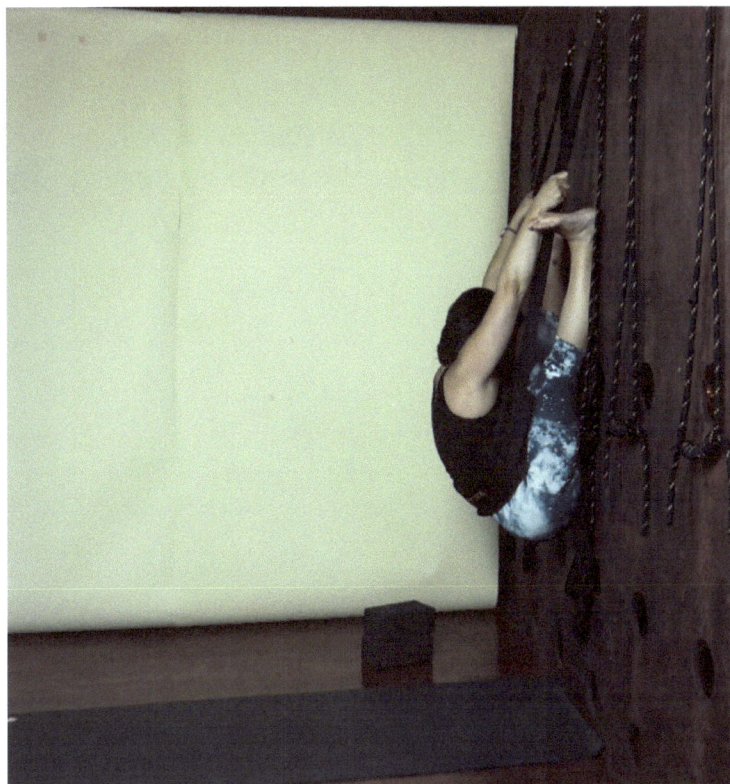

Lean back slightly,put your feet on the wall (knees wider and still outside of the straps) and push out, walking down like a mountain climber.

If you'd rather not try this yet, **check out the post under Child's Pose** and take the hanging version mentioned at the bottom of that post.

Hanging Backbend

This one is not for the weak at heart and I do not recommend it to beginners, ever. Please only attempt this is you have been practicing or have a strong backbend practice. You may want to have a spotter.

Stand away from the wall facing it with the hips in the sling. Walk the knees up the wall to about hip height (they may side up a little) and allow the upper body to reach back, drawing the hands to the floor.

Once the hands are at the floor, walk them back and grab the low handles. Push into the knees and pull with the hands. If you are super flexible, you may be able to walk the hands up to the higher handles.

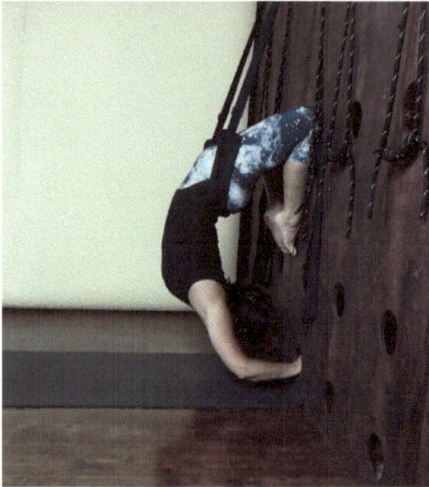

To come out, look up at your belly and reach the hands up to grab the sling, walking up and placing the feet down.

Here are just a couple other hanging poses that can be done. Turning round is a lesson for another day, but I leave these here for inspiration. Spiderwoman!

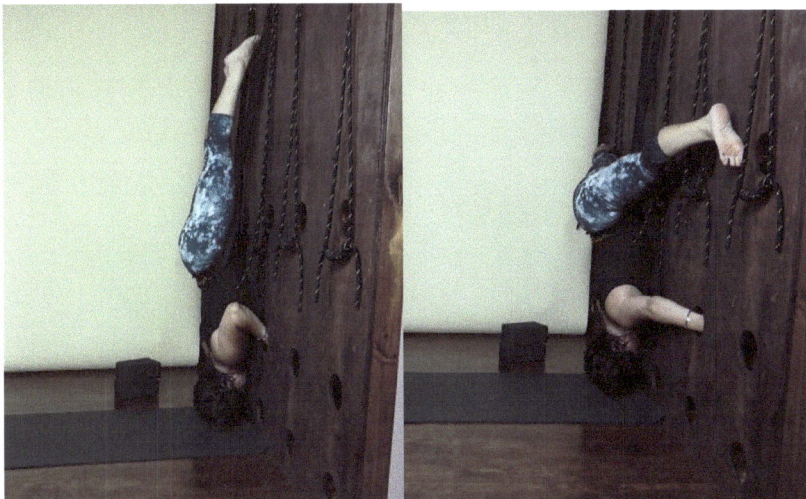

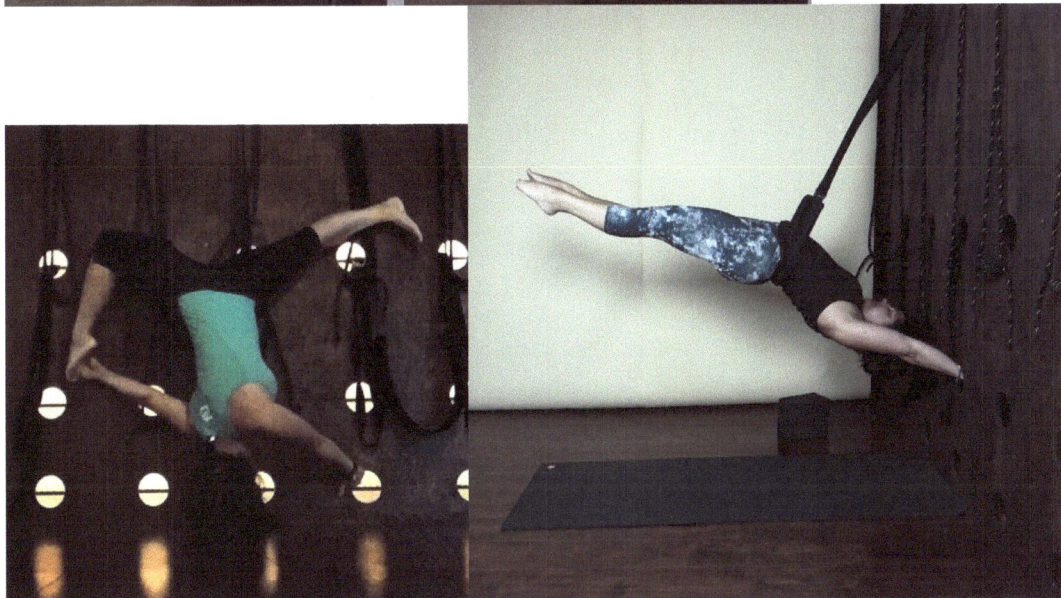

Hip Stretch Series

Hamstring Stretch

Stand with your back to the wall. Place your heel in the sling with the center of the heel in the center of the sling. Flex your toes towards you.

If you'd like to move on, hold the handles and gently slide your body forward to your point of resistance.

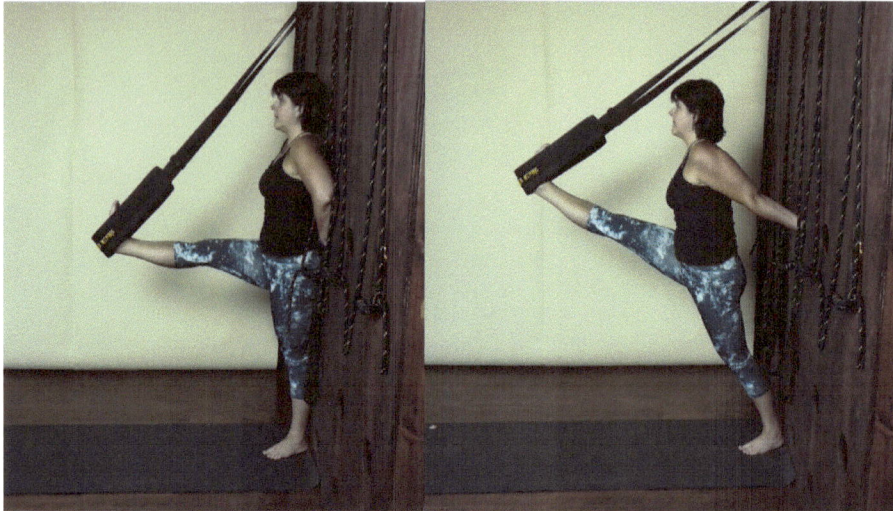

Pigeon

Turn your knee open (behind the strap) and put your foot in the sling on it's side. Lean forward over the bent leg.

If you'd like a deeper stretch, extend the foot away from you and lean into it just like in the hamstring stretch above. This stretch can be a suprisingly good alternative to pigeon for those with knee issues.

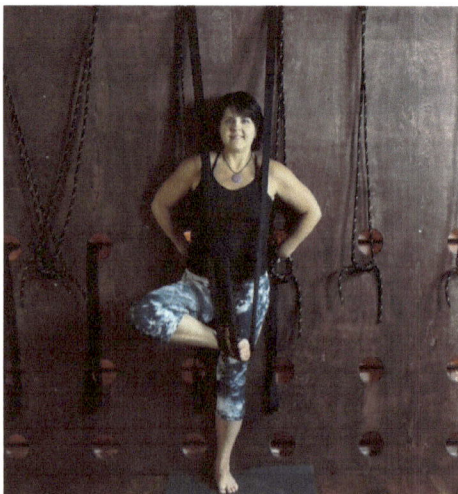

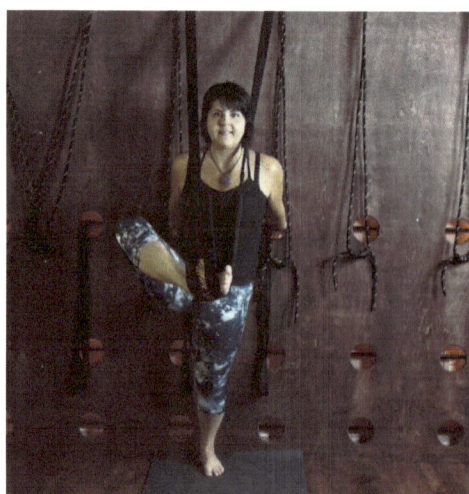

Side Leg Stretch.

Keeping the foot in the sling, if possible, turn to face the side, keeping the opposite hand on the handle at the wall for stability. Hold the sling with the free hand for conrol. Turn the toes and knee of the sling leg up towards the ceiling. Stay there, or gently slide out, holding the handles for staility. Work to move the hips forward and stay tall in the torso.

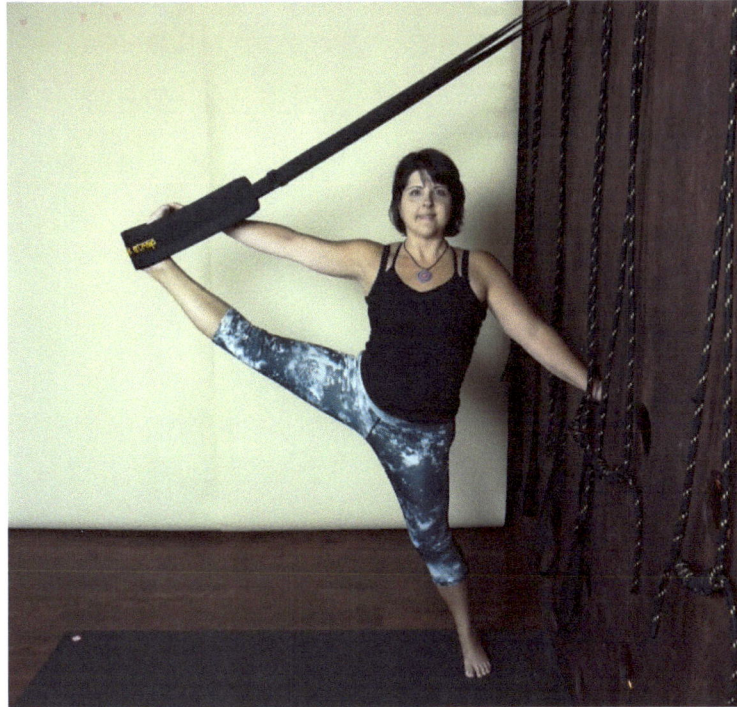

Bow into Down Dog Stretches and Handstand Prep

Standing Bow

Bring yourself to face the wall. Hold the handles and pull the sling out to the side. Make sure you haven't twisted the sling and slip it over your toes onto the ankle. Drop the knee down as you do this.

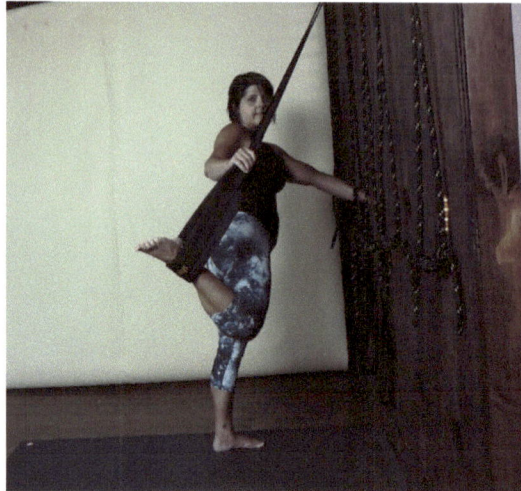

Bring both hands to the wall and begin to kick the leg back as you lift the chest up. It may also be nice to bring the chest to the wall and lift the arms up (not shown).

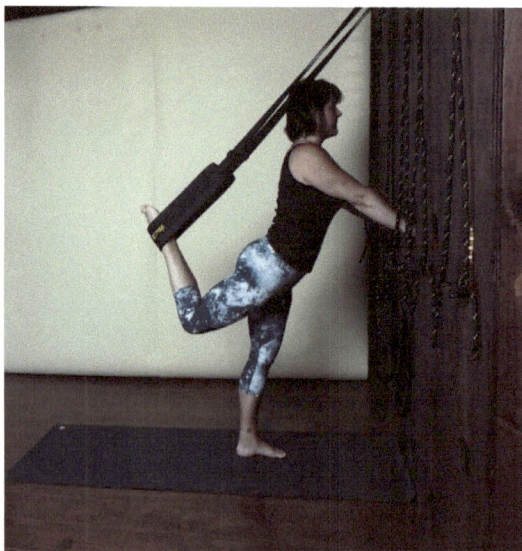

Eventually, you may hop back and kick the foot higher. Work to drop the sling leg's hip.

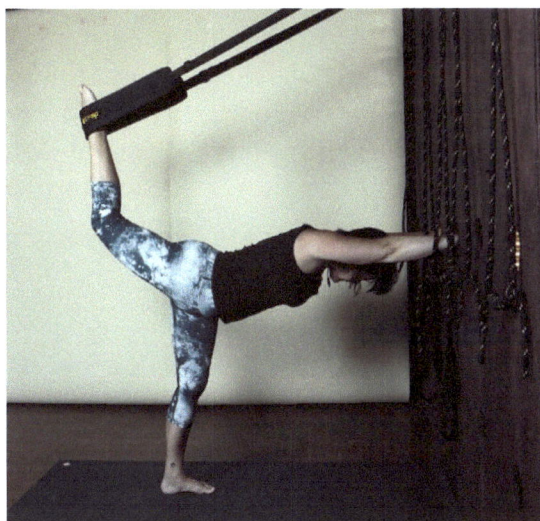

Walk the hands down, one handle at a time, staying at each position to feel it out. If you feel safe, walk the hands to the floor and step the floor foot back to a downward dog. Note: Sling height may need to be lowered for tighter hips.

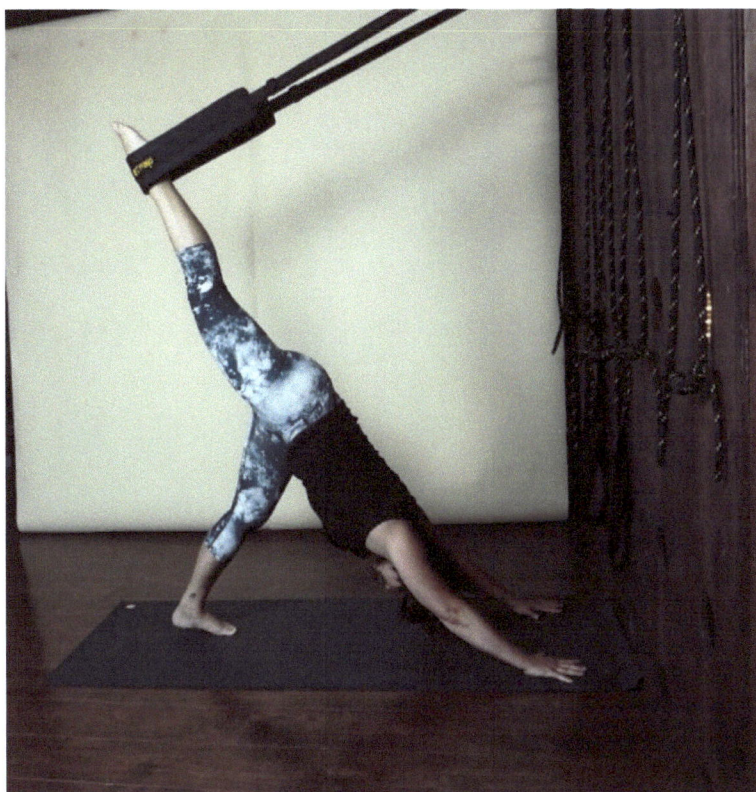

This next part takes tremendous strength and determination so approach it slowly. Press into the extended leg and see if you can lift the standing foor off the ground. *Start with lifing it just an inch and work up to lifting the knee into the chest. You MUST press down into the sling as well as the hands and lift out of the shoulders and the belly. Note: the sling may sway side to side so work with the test first!

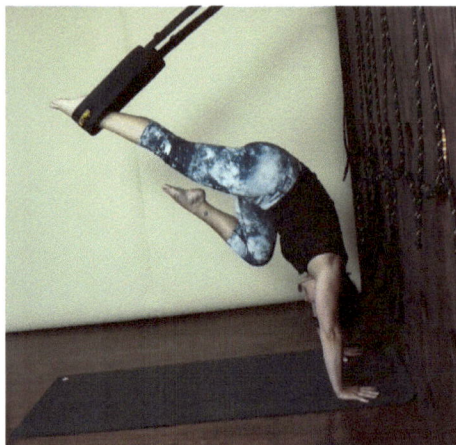

Once you feel you can do this securely, you may attempt to bring both feet into the sling by raising into the one legged lift, then slidnig the other leg into the sling. This takes a lot of arm, upper body and core strenth, so make sure you feel secure before proceeding.

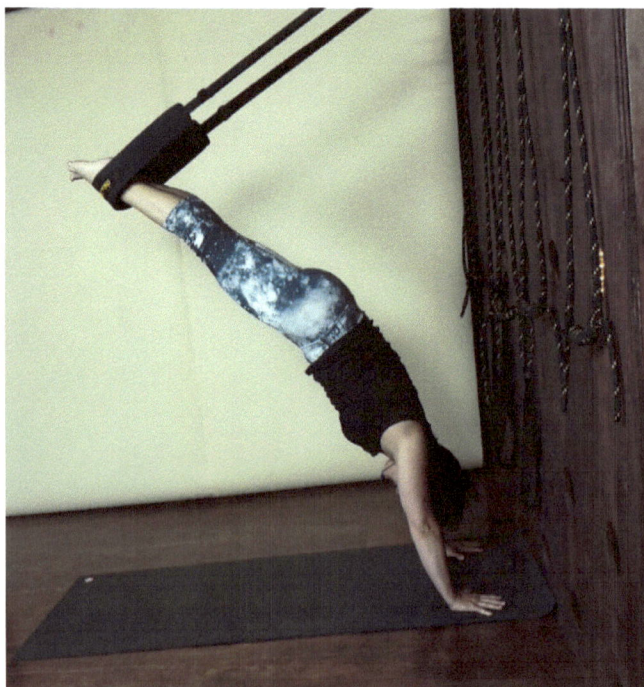

Next, work to pull the knees into the chest while lifting the hips up over the shoulders. Keep pressing into the sling or this will not work.

This exercise helps to develop strength and awareess for arm balances.

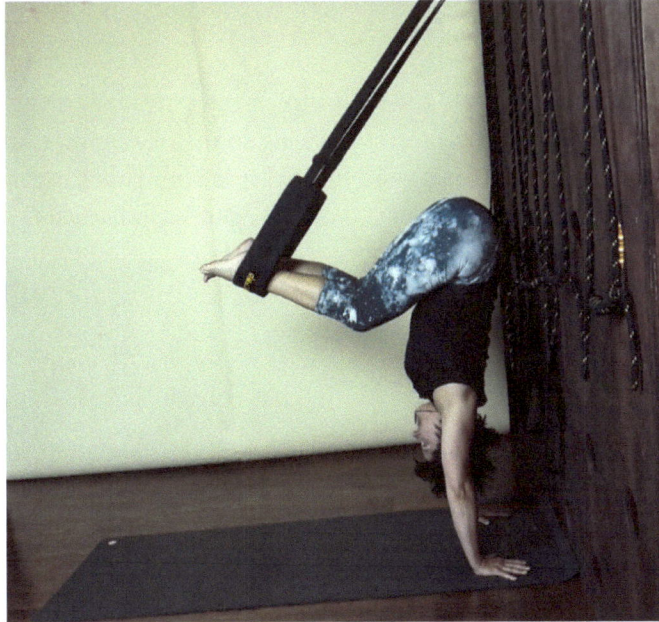

Once you are done, come back into a three legged downward dog then open the leg out to the side to get a nice inner thigh stretch.

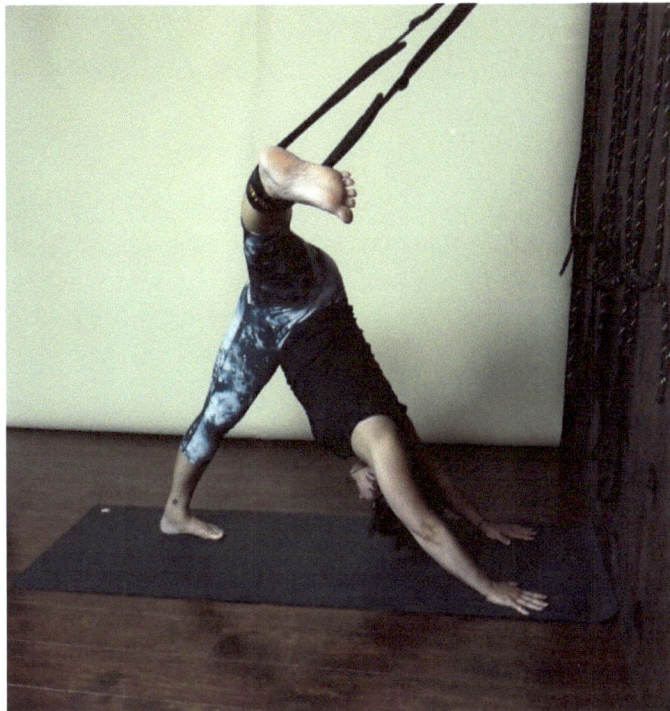

Sling Ankle Height

Lower the sling down to ankle height, just barely touching the floor.

There are only a few exercises we do at this height, and they are all quite restful and restorative.

Supported Bridge

Sit in front of the sling facing the wall. Hold the straps to lift the bottom and lower your shoulders to the floor in front of the sling. Lift your hips and adjust the sling so that it supports your hips. Your knees can be at the wall or you can place a block in between the wall and your knees. Having the knees rest on something will allow for a more restful pose. Rest your toes gently on the wall.

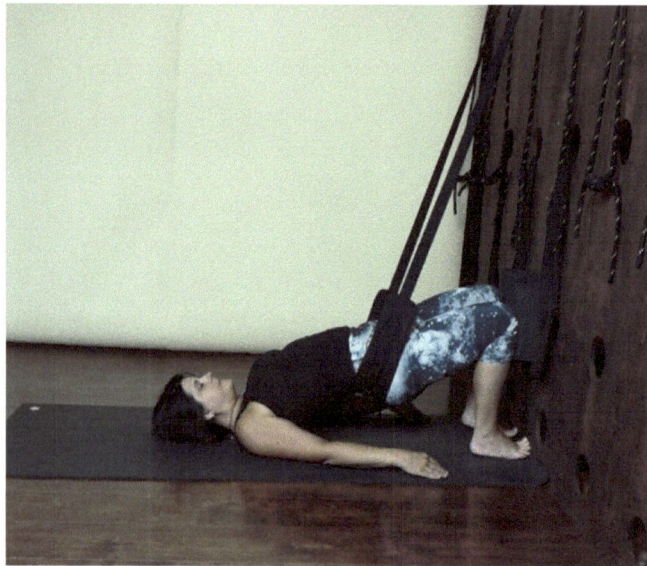

Legs Up the Wall Pose

Once you have been there for your alloted amount of time, release the blocks and hold the straps of the sling. Walk your feet up the wall and allow your bottom to slide to the wall.

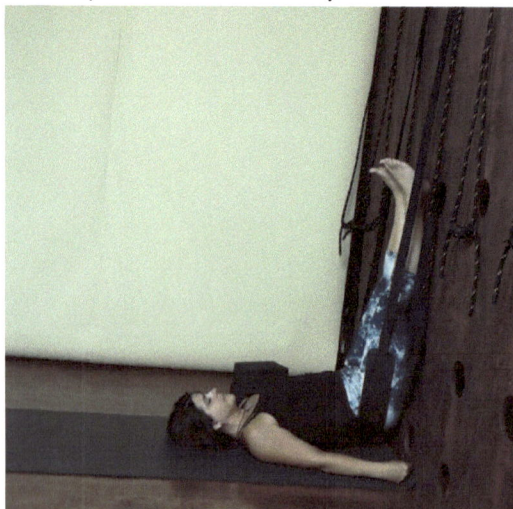

From Legs up the Wall, open your knees out and bring the souls of the feet together. You can leave them at the wall, but it is also nice to wrap them under and around the straps (not shown but as in the backward hanging version). We use this as our savasana, often.

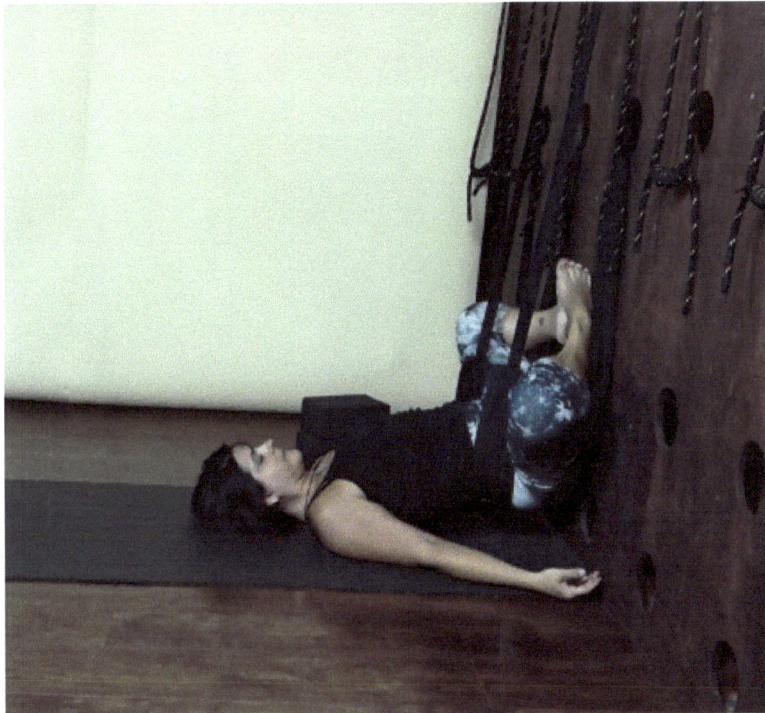

It can be nice to reach the arms overhead.

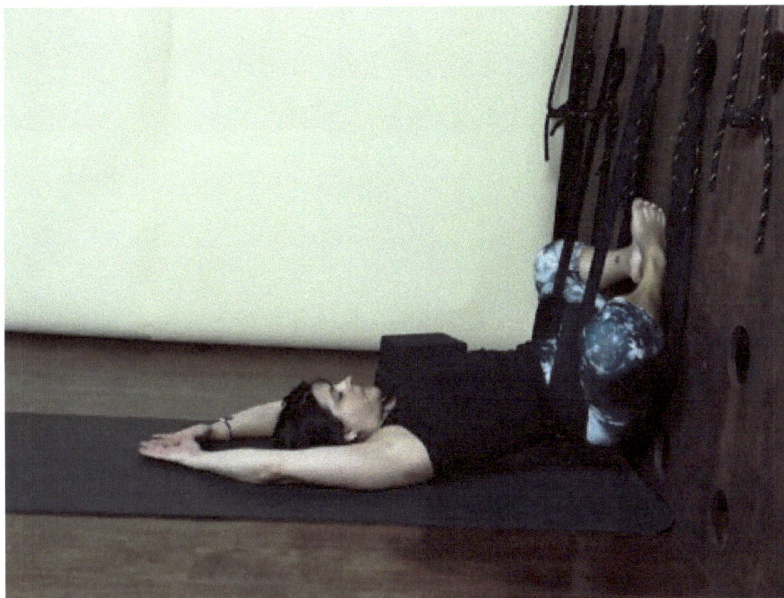

Neck Traction in Savasana

This is another favorite variation of savasana.

It is nice to have a bolster for your knees; however, it is not necessary.

Lay with your head to the wall and move about a foot or so from it. Place the sling around the base of your skull. Move out until you feel the traction, however not far enough that the sling slides off the head.

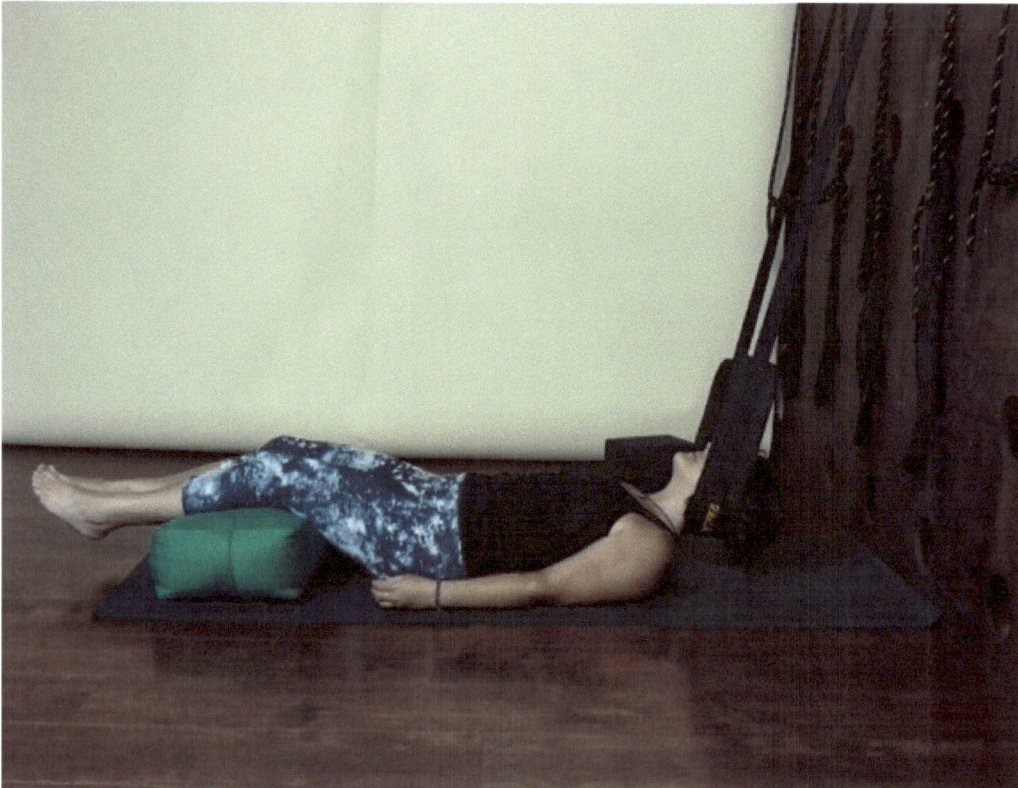

A few things I've played with put here for inspiration – there are no limits except those we accept.

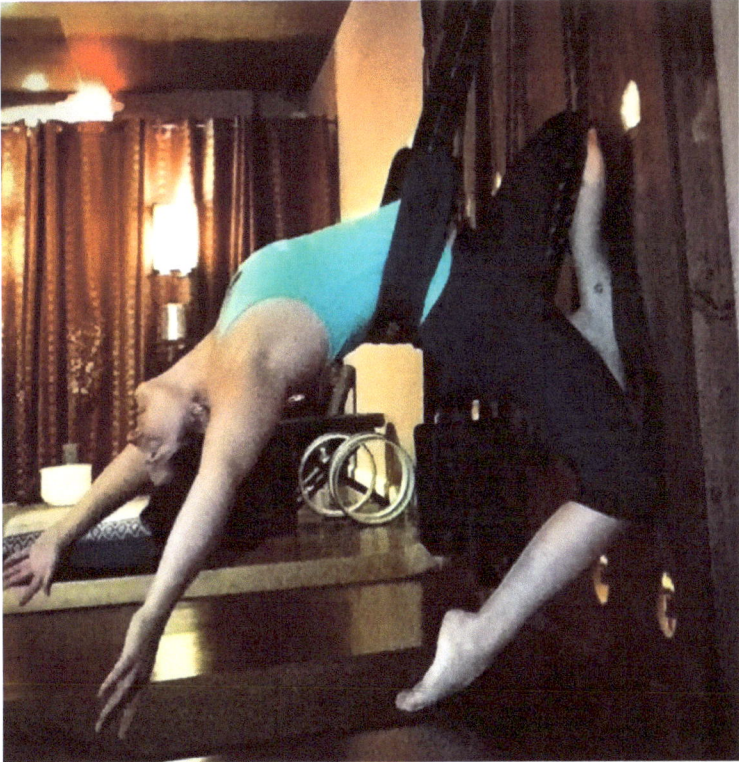

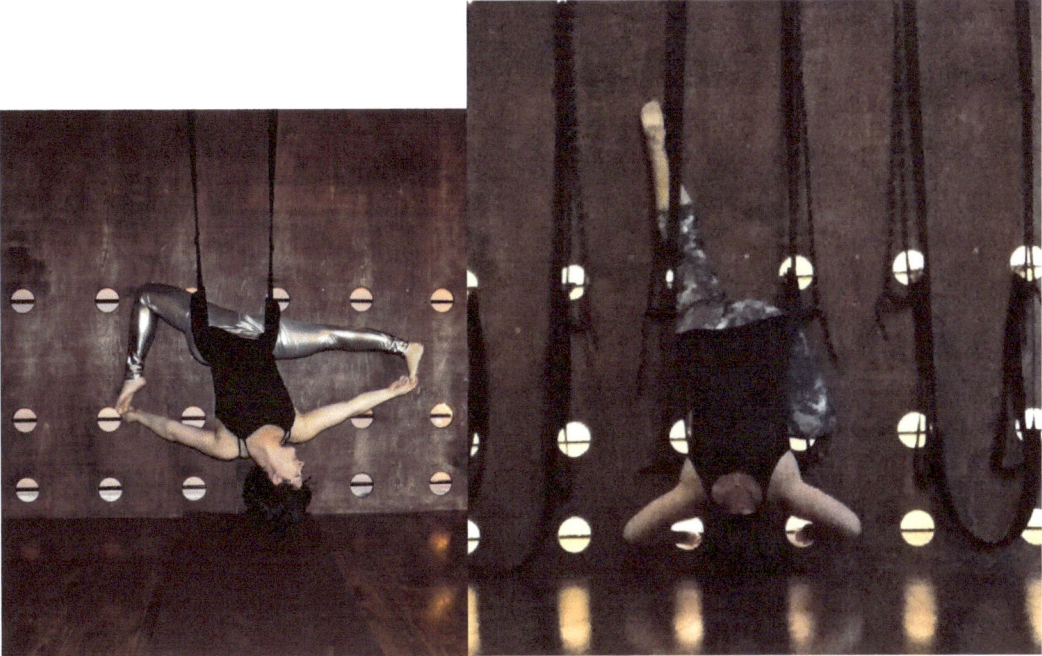

These final words which I hope will make some sense and help you stay safe in your practice.

The practice is acceptance, for without it we fail.

Being able to say "My body is not ready to go there, today." (and accept that), is the first step in finding a way past the obstacles. An alcoholic must first admit he is an alcoholic before he can begin to move past it. The same applies to all things.

Accept, then do the work.

I hope you have found this book helpful on your journey.

Namaste.

Photographs taken by Jeremy Spitzberg

About the Author

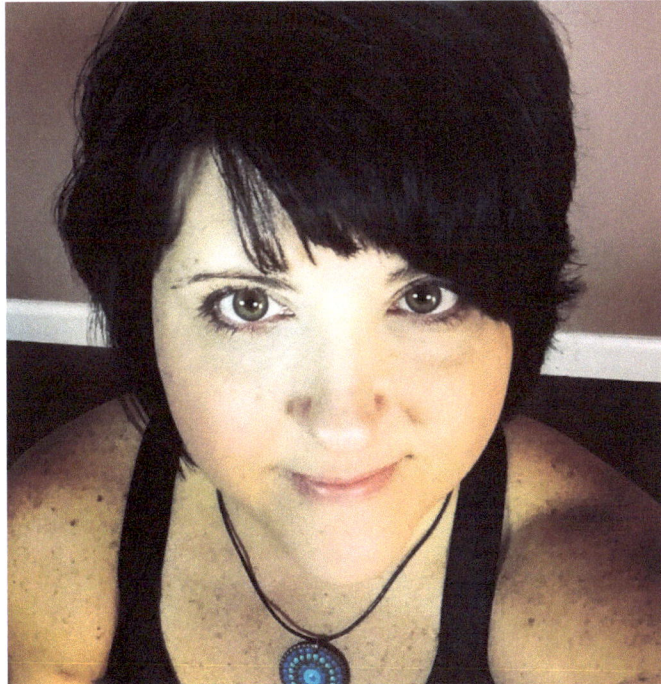

Deanna Aliano

Deanna is a dedicated holistic health practitioner. She began her training as a massage therapist, learning anatomy, physiology and biomechanics. She was trained as a full Pilates instructor, offering individual sessions and classes on the main Pilates training equipment and mat. She is trained in Thai Yoga massage and has practiced it for 15 years.

Her journey into yoga began while taking Iyengar based classes, which appealed to her because of the strong attention to alignment and modifications. She went on to study various forms of yoga, including Asthanga, Viniyoga, Sivinanda, Bikram, Kripalu and Baptiste before she decided to do her teacher training with Sri Dharma Mittra in New York. She has studied with Allison West, Sadie Nardini, Todd Norian, Raji Thron, Street Yoga, and more, and is proud to be a certified AiRealYoga teacher under Carmen Curtis.

Deanna specializes in teaching asana practice with a high degree of alignment and attention to the core, while infusing fun and lightheartedness into the practice.

Deanna is available for workshops, trainings and talks. Please contact her via
DeannaDYoga@gmail.com.

Follow @DeannaDYoga on Instagram and Vimeo for free mini classes on technique. Full classes are also available.

www.ingramcontent.com/pod-product-compliance
Lightning Source LLC
Chambersburg PA
CBHW060821270326
41931CB00002B/43